LABOR PAIN:
WHAT'S *YOUR* BEST STRATEGY?

Get the Data.
Make a Plan.
Take Charge of Your Birth.

Henci Goer

The Take Charge of Your Birth Series

An S Press Book

Published by S Press

Copyright 2022 by Henci Goer. All rights reserved.

Book design by Merlin Andrews

Cover design by Hannah Gaskamp

Illustrations by Emily Jaksa

Photography by Adobe Stock (jbrown), Growing Wings Photography, Tyler Olson, and Wirthy Photography. Photograph of author by Chris Shum Photography.

Reading Labor Pain: What's *Your* Best Strategy? *is like having a conversation with a wise, knowledgeable, caring friend. Goer presents pain relief options and then, simply but in great depth, the evidence-based benefits and risks of each option. Like a trusted friend she emphasizes that decisions on managing labor pain are personal. A must-read for not only childbearing women but for those who care for them!*

Judith Lothian, RN, PhD, LCCE, FAAN; Associate Editor *Journal of Perinatal Education*; Co-author of *Giving Birth with Confidence*

Henci's superpower is taking super-detailed (and frankly boring!) birth evidence and translating it into something easily understood by parents. This book is no exception! She gives you the information you need in a straightforward and approachable way, and then she walks you through the pros and cons of each option. In our years as doulas we've seen that women rarely receive all the information they need in order to make an informed decision. No more! This little book gives you everything you need to keep your power and make decisions that are best for your body, your birth and your baby. Well done, Henci!

Alicia & Meredith; Childbirth Educators; IntentionalBirth.co

Henci has always impressed me with her intellect, knowledge, wisdom, humor, and writing skills. I'm thrilled these gifts will be available to readers in her Take Charge of Your Birth *series.*

Penny Simkin, PT; Co-founder of DONA International; Co-author of *Pregnancy, Childbirth & the Newborn*; Author of *The Birth Partner*

She has done it again! The author has synthesized the current data on the various strategies for getting through labor with the joy of birth intact. Her critical analysis is thick with data to support her position, yet it is presented in a balanced and readable form—with lots of opportunity for those who want to "dive deep" into the scientific literature if they wish, as they become increasingly sophisticated about their upcoming birth. Thus, it's a book to read and re-read before birth, and even after your birth as you prepare for your possible next.

Michael C. Klein CM, MD, FCFP, CCFP, FAAP (neonatal-perinatal); Emeritus Professor, Family Practice & Pediatrics, University of British Columbia; Sr. Scientist Emeritus, BC Children's Hospital Research Institute, Vancouver; Author of *Dissident Doctor—Catching Babies and Challenging the Medical Status Quo*

Henci Goer, a trusted advocate for women's autonomy in childbirth, shares her wealth of knowledge in this judgment-free, easy-to-read guide to labor pain. Pregnant people and their support networks will find valuable, fact-based information to help them make sense of the research on coping with labor pain. As the series title implies, this book will empower women with data to confidently take charge of their births.

Joyce K. Edmonds, PhD, MPH, RN; Editor-in-Chief JOGNN (*Journal of Obstetric, Gynecologic, & Neonatal Nursing*)

I have long been an admirer of Henci Goer. Henci's understanding of the complexities of the culture of maternity care in the USA and how these issues interlink with what we do and don't know about obstetric interventions is unparalleled. Henci explains the issues and the evidence with clarity, honesty, and humour. She offers summaries AND depth, depending on what you need, and encourages you to make the decisions that are right for you. This book is a great resource for your birth planning toolkit.

Dr. Sara Wickham, PhD, RM, BA(Hons), MA, PGCert.; Midwife, Author, Speaker; Researcher and Director of the Birth Information Project at www.sarawickham.com

Henci Goer has done it again! This book is not just for expecting moms; it's for the entire birth team. As a doula and childbirth educator, I am constantly in awe of Henci's ability to present evidence in a nonjudgmental way. I'll be recommending this book with zero hesitation to all of my clients and students for years to come.

Kyleigh Banks; Founder of Birthworker.com

Dedicated to Harriet Palmer, CNM,
midwife and educator extraordinaire.
She taught me much, and she was my friend.
May her memory be a blessing.

Table of
Contents

Preface

B efore we sit down together, I thought you might like to know a little more about me and why I've written this book. You can, of course, get my qualifications for writing it from my bio, but I mean something a bit more personal.

My Story

My passion and my life's work have been providing pregnant women what they need to make decisions about their care: complete and accurate information, presented neutrally, on the pros and cons of all their options.

My passion arose from my experience of my first two births. Both were medically uneventful vaginal births to a healthy baby. At both births, my caregivers were competent and everyone was nice to me. Nonetheless, I emerged from the first birth feeling distressed, defeated, and diminished, lacking confidence in myself and my body. In contrast, after my second birth, I felt exhilarated, proud, and strong. What, then, was the difference?

At the first birth in 1974, I assumed my caregivers knew better than I what was right for me and everything they did had to be for the best. I was persuaded to have an opioid injection for pain even though my Lamaze techniques were working for me and I wasn't feeling the need for pain meds. All I got from it was a losing battle to surface from my drugged haze to try to cope with contractions. I remember trying to push lying flat on my back and pleading that if I could just sit up more, I could push more forcefully. I was ignored. After pushing awhile longer to little effect, I ended up with a large *episiotomy*—cutting the vaginal opening to enlarge it for birth—and a forceps delivery. I desperately wanted to be with my baby, but after just a few minutes to hold him, he was taken away for a routine twelve hours of observation in the nursery. Because he was born at noon, he wasn't brought to me again until the next morning. At that point, hurting from the episiotomy and the forceps delivery, feeling exhausted and overwhelmed, the best I could work up was that I thought he was cute. It took weeks to heal from the delivery, and sadly, I went on feeling no more emotion for my son than a sense of duty toward him for months after his birth.

I put my difficulties down to my inadequacies. That's where things stood until my next pregnancy two years later when I started considering what I wanted and didn't want for this next birth. As I began reading and exploring, I found that none of the practices and policies that had caused me such physical and emotional pain had been necessary in my case. All had been avoidable. If only I had known …

This time, I sought out a care provider who saw me as an active contributor: someone with concerns, insights, and judgments to be respected as much as his own. As a result, my second birth experience couldn't have been more different, although it was the more difficult labor. My daughter was in *occiput posterior* position, a situation where the baby is facing the mother's belly instead of her back. Babies may not be able to descend through the pelvis until they turn into the more favorable *occiput anterior* position, and sometimes the malposition causes the mother excruciating back pain, which it did in my case.

In this birth, though, I was supported and encouraged in my desire for an unmedicated birth. When I got to pushing, my doctor recommended that I push on my hands and knees so that gravity could assist the baby in turning to face my back. As I did so, he used his hand to gently help bring her head around. Once she swiveled into the anterior position, I easily pushed her out in a very few contractions with no episiotomy, despite her weighing one and a half pounds more than her brother. Once she was born, she came immediately to my arms and was in my arms or my husband's arms for the first couple of hours after her birth except for a brief examination. I felt on top of the world, thrilled with myself, and instantly in love with my baby.

Here's what those two births taught me: when it comes to how you feel afterward, it's far less about how easy or difficult the labor and birth were or whether everything went according to your preferences or how you imagined it would; it's far more about whether you participated in the decisions, you made the ultimate calls, and your caregivers listened to and respected you. And yes, I subsequently found research that agrees with that.

By the time my daughter was a few months old, I realized I wanted to share with other women what I had learned about the importance of having agency in the decisions that are made during labor and birth. I joined a group that was opening a birth-resources center and founding a community-owned and -operated freestanding birth center. I began working as a doula (there were no formal training programs for doulas yet) at the birth center and trained as a Lamaze teacher, all in the interest of wanting women to know that they have choices and the right to make them, and that having their autonomy respected matters to how they feel about themselves, their babies, and their partners.

Eventually, I realized there are many excellent birth educators and doulas, and I could fill a niche that was less crowded and had the potential to reach more people: I could read, analyze, and synthesize the obstetric research. It's not that difficult, really. All it requires is having college-level reading skills, acquiring the specialized vocabulary, understanding statistical concepts, and being able to think critically. Very few people, then or today, though, were engaged in that task. So I shifted gears, and that's what I've been doing for the last thirty-five years and counting. This book is my latest project.

Enough about me. Let's turn to you, now, and how I think I can be of help.

Why This Book?

This book, as does all my work over the years, has one purpose: I want you to learn the easy way what I learned the hard way. I don't want you to find yourself thinking later: "I never knew that was an option. If I had, I would have gone for it," or "If I had known that could happen, I would have made a different choice." The book's subtitle—*Get the Data. Make a Plan. Take Charge of Your Birth.*—sums up my ideas on how best to accomplish that goal. Let me take you through the sequence step by step.

To begin with, if you're going to make a choice, you need to get the data—meaning, as I said above, complete, accurate, fact-based information on the pros and cons of all your options. Getting data, as opposed to opinions, can be difficult. Whether they practice standard obstetric management or favor refraining from medical intervention whenever possible, many of the birth professionals you would expect to be your source for data are convinced they know what you should choose. Consequently, they may consciously or unconsciously tell you only as much as they think you need to know to persuade you to do what they think is best. Friends, relatives, and media sources have opinions, and while other people's thoughts, feelings, and experiences can be valuable, they aren't data either.

This is where I hope to help. This book will present the research evidence in a digestible format so that you can decide for yourself. And while that will involve interpretation on my part, which introduces my judgment, I will compensate for that by playing my cards face up. I will always tell you why I think what I think about the evidence. I also promise to stick to reasoned analysis and avoid loaded language that evokes strong feelings that may override your thought processes.

Once you've taken in the data, the next step is to make a plan, that is, to decide what's right for you and what you can do to maximize your chances of getting it. More than a few birth professionals, though, find birth plans problematic. They think making a plan leads women to think they can control an uncontrollable process, a mindset likely to end in frustration, disappointment, and even feelings of failure when they find out they can't. Best not to make choices, they say, and just go with the flow.

They are right if you think of a plan as a shopping list or blueprint. However, that's a narrow conception of what a plan can be. Planning for a birth is more like planning a vacation or a career. It's the same process of using heart (values, inner knowing) and head (information gathering, practical considerations) to figure out what you want and what best promotes getting it. Certainly, obstacles may crop up, but if they do, knowing what's important to you, where you're headed, and the route you're taking will help you navigate, adapt, and modify. And, should things really go sideways, you'll be prepared to take a different direction while salvaging what can be salvaged of your plan.

A plan is a crucial element of having agency, and having agency, as I said, matters profoundly. Feeling strong and capable (or the reverse) as you encounter the challenges of new motherhood affects not just you but also your baby and other members of your family. A malleable plan will serve you far better than drifting with the tide and letting others decide what's best for you. I can help you with your plan as well. In addition to providing the data, I can give you ideas and suggestions for bringing your plan to fruition and avoiding common pitfalls.

Finally, having a plan based on the data enables you to take charge of your birth. Notice I didn't say "control." You can't control the birth—or, really, anything in life. You can, though, take charge by knowing what you want and why, then planning how best to achieve it. Having said all that, I want to add that you can, of course, decide to leave a decision up to your care provider or simply follow their recommendation. I just want you to make that decision consciously and not because you didn't think you could do anything different. Also, by knowing what you want, you'll be able to choose care providers who are in alignment with you and whose judgment you can trust.

So let's set out on your journey together. I'm here as a resource to help you find your own path. If something I tell you resonates with you, great! If

LABOR PAIN: WHAT'S YOUR BEST STRATEGY?

something doesn't feel right for you, that's OK too. Figuring out what you don't want is as useful as figuring out what you do want. Take what works for you in this book and leave the rest behind. Trust yourself. You have what you need to decide what's best for you, and I've got your back.

Chapter 1:
Introduction

If you are pregnant, or even thinking about becoming pregnant, chances are labor pain has crossed your mind. And if you've been looking into your options, odds are you've been hearing all the reasons to make epidurals "Plan A" from your doctor, your friends, and on social media. But only hearing the positives about one of your options isn't the best way to make a decision on any important issue. I think you are better served by hearing about the advantages and disadvantages of *all* your options so you can make the decision that's right for you. I intend to provide that in this book.

As you may have already discovered, though, people generally have strong opinions on how best to deal with labor pain. The truth is that no one with an interest in the subject can be completely objective. They may try, but what they choose to present and how they frame it will inevitably be colored by their own thoughts, beliefs, and experiences. Objectivity simply isn't attainable.

That truth, though, raises another question: How can I fairly represent your options to you if no one, including me, can be completely neutral? I gave this much thought in the planning and writing of this book, and the answer is: transparency.

One aspect of transparency is to be explicit about my opinions so you know exactly where I stand. So let's start with that.

- I believe the best person to decide what is right for you is you.

- I believe an epidural can be a godsend for some labors.

- I also believe that because of their many potential adverse effects, as with any medical intervention, epidurals are best reserved for situations when lesser measures have failed and the benefits outweigh the risks.

- I believe NO ONE has the right to dictate to another person where their "enough" point is when it comes to pain, nor may they judge them for where they draw the line.

- I believe that working with labor pain using non-drug strategies alone can have its rewards.

- I also believe that deciding to pursue those rewards is a purely personal choice, and no one should judge another person for what pain-relief methods they choose.

The rest of being transparent is in the writing of the book itself. Transparency is why I give you the actual data and its source. That way, you'll have the facts, not just my interpretation of them. Transparency is also why, when I discuss controversial issues, I won't just tell you what I think but why I think it. That way you can form your own judgments. Finally, in the few places where I express an opinion, I'll be very clear that's what I'm doing. Making that distinction will allow you to assign the proper weight to what I'm saying.

OK. I've told you about my intent for this book and explained how I will, to the best of my ability, give you what you need to decide what's best for you free of pressure in any direction. Now let's turn to its structure.

ABOUT THE BOOK

Chapters 2 through 6 will go through each of your labor-coping options and discuss:

- what's involved in obtaining it,

- how well it relieves pain,

- its advantages, and

- its disadvantages and adverse effects according to the medical research, including how likely adverse effects are to occur.

The chapters are meant to be read independently, so start with any pain-relief method that interests you.

The epidural chapter and the chapter on non-drug options, which I've dubbed "DIY strategies," have a bonus section at the end titled "Taking a Deeper Dive." The Deeper Dive is where we'll discuss the details of particularly complex information that may be of interest to some, but not all, readers. If you just want the data you need to make a decision, feel free to skip the bonus sections; they are there for those who are interested in … well, taking a deeper dive.

The chapters covering pain-relief options should give you a full enough picture to make up your mind about whether the pros outweigh the cons or vice versa for any given strategy. However, you also need practical strategies for carrying out your plans. For this reason, Chapter 7, "Your Take-Away," is a collection of ideas, suggestions, and tips that should prove helpful in implementing your plan for coping with labor pain, whatever that plan may be.

As you read through and consider your options, keep in mind that you don't have to feel married to a particular choice. You may make a plan you think will be a good fit, then change your mind during labor; I'll help with that, too. Should that switch be from planning an unmedicated birth to having an epidural, the "Take-Away" chapter will include suggestions for how to manage the switch in a way that will facilitate feeling good about your decision.

I end the book with a chapter in which I offer my opinion. I put this chapter last because I wanted you to have my opinion in case it's of interest to you, but I wanted you to have it after having the opportunity to make up your own mind first, unswayed by me.

Finally, the book wraps up with a comparison table across all the methods for dealing with labor pain covered in the book. The table will enable you to see at a glance how they stack up against each other with respect to:

- degree of pain relief,

- lag time to pain relief,

- effect on consciousness or psychological state,

- cost,

- side effects,

- effect on mode of delivery,

- effect on the baby,

- severe/life-threatening effects, and

- miscellaneous problems.

My hope is that this book will provide you everything you need to decide on your best strategy for coping with labor pain, to be able to reassess in labor if you need to, and to feel good about your birth experience after-ward—in other words, to take charge of your birth.

Chapter 2:
Epidurals

As I wrote in the introductory chapter, epidural analgesia is the main item on the menu of coping options for labor pain, so odds are it's the one you've been thinking about most. It makes sense, then, to tackle epidurals first.

Again, I have no investment in what choice you make, but I want you to make it with eyes open, knowing the pros and cons of all your options. For this reason, I'll devote a full chapter to each pain-coping method that covers what's involved, how well it relieves pain, and detailed information on its advantages and disadvantages.

Accordingly, let's get started with what you need to know about epidurals, beginning with what's involved in administering one.

6

WHAT'S INVOLVED IN ADMINISTERING AN EPIDURAL?

EPIDURAL PREP

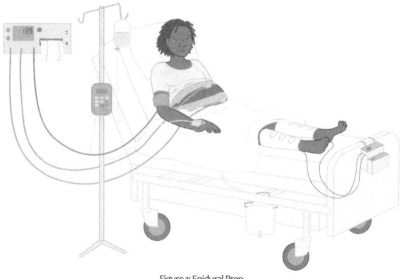

Figure 1: Epidural Prep

Figure 1 illustrates the components of the epidural prep. To prepare for an epidural, the nurse starts an IV and administers a *bolus* of fluid (a substantial amount—usually one liter, or about a quart—over a short period of time) to try to prevent a drop in blood pressure, a common epidural side effect.

The nurse places a blood-pressure cuff so blood pressure can be closely monitored. The cuff is usually automated. It periodically inflates and deflates, transmitting its data to the central nursing station.

Belts are placed around your abdomen with leads to a fetal monitor. The upper belt's sensor picks up each labor contraction, and the lower belt's sensor uses ultrasound to pick up the baby's heart rate. This data is transmitted to the central nursing station as well, letting nurses know if the epidural is having adverse effects on the fetal heart rate.

The epidural prevents the ability to urinate, so a catheter may be passed through the urethra into the bladder and left there to keep it drained, or this procedure may be performed periodically.

In many hospitals, your legs are wrapped in intermittent-compression cuffs that rhythmically inflate and deflate to help pump blood through them as a preventative for deep venous clots, a potential result of being mostly immobile for many hours.

EPIDURAL ADMINISTRATION

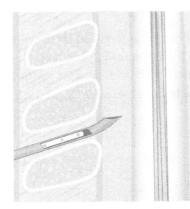

Figure 2: Epidural Needle Insertion

Figures 2 and 3 illustrate the details of the actual procedure. To orient you, you're looking at a side view. The oblong shapes stacked vertically on the left depict the spinal vertebrae seen in cross section. The tube on the right is the dural membrane, which sheathes the spinal cord. The spinal cord—or more specifically at this level of the back, the bundle of nerves that emerges from the base of the spinal column—is shown as a darker column in the center of the tube.

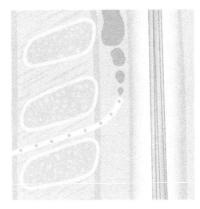

Figure 3: Epidural Catheter Delivering Anesthetic

To administer the epidural, you are asked to sit up or lie on one side with your back curled. After your back is washed with antiseptic and draped, the anesthesiologist (or nurse anesthetist) injects a local anesthetic to numb the skin. Then they slip a needle between the spinal vertebrae of the lower back into a space just to the outside (*epi*) of the membrane (*dura*) that wraps the spinal cord, hence the name epidural. Next, the anesthesiologist performs tests to make sure the needle isn't accidentally in a blood vessel or hasn't pierced the dura into the space beneath, either of which can cause life-threatening complications. If everything checks out, the anesthesiologist inserts a tiny, flexible plastic tube (*catheter*) through the needle into the space, withdraws the needle, and tapes the catheter to your back. A mixture of anesthetic—a drug in the same family that dentists use—and opioid is then injected into the catheter.

Anesthesia can be maintained in several different ways. (See Figures 4–6.) The catheter can be attached to a pump that slowly administers a *continuous* dose or to a pump that permits you to self-administer a pre-measured dose as you feel the need (*patient-controlled analgesia*). Less commonly these days, it may be maintained by the anesthesiologist coming in periodically to administer another dose via the catheter (these doses are called *top-ups*).

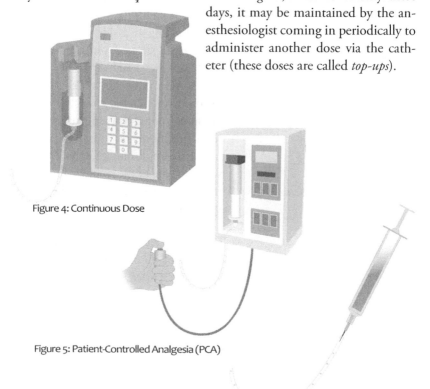

Figure 4: Continuous Dose

Figure 5: Patient-Controlled Analgesia (PCA)

Figure 6: Periodic Top-Ups

How Well Do Epidurals Relieve Pain?

The goal of a labor epidural is to completely relieve pain while still allowing you to feel some sensation and have some motor function. The advantage of that balance is that you can move your legs and know when to push. Sometimes, though, coverage can be patchy, and sometimes the epidural doesn't "take" on one side or at all. Depending on the study, 7 to 9 percent of women rated epidurals as "not very helpful" or "not helpful at all." [22, 29, 54]

What Are an Epidural's Advantages?

Epidurals offer several advantages:

1. **They are the only strategy capable of completely relieving pain.**

2. **They allow women to be awake and aware.** Unlike IV or muscular injections of opioids, which we'll get to in Chapter 4, epidurals don't dull consciousness.

3. **They permit rest or sleep.** Because of how effectively they can relieve pain, they can offer respite from a difficult or prolonged labor.

4. **Women report that having an epidural enabled them to focus outwardly, which allowed them to relax, engage with the people around them, and enjoy the birth.** [5, 66]

5. **Anecdotally, they can sometimes put a stalled labor back on track.** While epidurals generally slow labor, sometimes they have the opposite effect. The theory is that the complete muscle relaxation they induce can sometimes release whatever is holding up progress.

WHAT ARE AN EPIDURAL'S DISADVANTAGES?

Now we come to the disadvantages of epidurals. This section is going to be much longer than the section on the advantages because, as you may have gathered from what's involved in administering one, epidurals have wide-ranging effects. The fact that this is so, I should add, in no way undercuts their advantages.

Laying out the issues for you also presents a challenge. An epidural's advantages are simple and straightforward, but explaining their disadvantages is often neither, mostly for reasons having to do with the limitations of the research studying them. (See "Problems with the Research" in "Taking a Deeper Dive.") That poses a dilemma. If I lay out the reasoning behind everything I'm about to say about the downside of epidurals, I risk your eyes glazing over from information overload. But if I just give you a simplified version, then you've only got my word for it, and I want you to be able to make your own judgments as to whether I've made my case—especially since in some instances, I'll be at odds with conventional wisdom.

I decided the solution is to let you choose your own adventure. That way, you can decide how deep you want to go.

Here's the plan:

In this section of this chapter, I'll give you a numbered list of epidural disadvantages along with a brief explanation for each one, giving you the basic information needed to make an informed choice. If you see a diamond in the margin and the phrase "Taking a Deeper Dive," that means additional information is available in "Taking a Deeper Dive" at the end of this chapter. If you want to find out more, you can go to the "Deeper Dive" to find the corresponding number and diamond. There, you'll read a more detailed discussion of the issues and research and sometimes an explanation of why epidurals have a particular adverse effect.

Hopefully, this setup will enable you to investigate further quickly and easily when you wish.

One more important point: Remember I said the research had weaknesses? Well, the cumulative result of those weaknesses is that *much of what is commonly accepted as undisputed Truth about what epidurals do and don't do is a best-case scenario and probably not accurate.* (If you want to know my grounds for that statement, you'll find it under "Problems with the Research" in "Taking a Deeper Dive.") To tip you off to instances where this may be the case, I'll use **maximum** and **minimum** to differentiate when the odds of experiencing an adverse effect may be greater than they appear.

Oh, and just so you know, in the "Take-Away" chapter later in this book, I'll be giving you a list of strategies for reducing the probability and impact of epidural adverse effects.

OK. Here, then, is the list of epidural disadvantages:

1. **Having an epidural may increase your out-of-pocket costs for the birth.** Out-of-pocket epidural costs may range as high as three thousand dollars even if you have insurance.[15, 21]

◊ 2. **Epidurals convert birth into a medical process controlled by medical staff.** Planning an epidural means ascribing to the medical model of childbirth. Within this model, birth is viewed as a solely physical and potentially pathological process. Accordingly, the aim becomes to deliver a baby as efficiently and painlessly as possible, relying on close monitoring and frequent or routine use of medications and procedures to accomplish that goal. The *experience* of birth, other than as it relates to pain control, is no more than a minor consideration in this model. There is, however, another model—physiologic care—in which labor is viewed as a normal physiologic process and a significant life event requiring no more than supportive care for most women and only turning to medical management for more medically complex labors. This model engages with the woman as a birth giver and care takes into account the emotional, psychological, and spiritual aspects of childbirth. (I explain more about this model in "Taking a Deeper Dive.")

3. **Epidurals have a long delay between request and relief.** It can easily take an hour to get the bolus of IV fluid on board, get prepped for the procedure, have the epidural administered, and have it reach full effect—and that's if the anesthesiologist is readily available.

4. **Epidurals require a package of practices intended to prevent, monitor for, and counteract the epidural's potential adverse effects.** The package includes an IV and a large amount of IV fluid as part of the epidural prep; continuous monitoring of the baby's heart rate and mother's contraction strength; and bladder catheterization. It also includes a high probability of being given IV oxytocin (aka Pitocin or "Pit" and Syntocinon) to strengthen contractions. All the items in the package have potential adverse effects as well as benefits.

◊ 5. **Epidurals can have unpleasant side effects.** These include:

   • **Nausea or vomiting.** A minimum of 10 percent of women who have an epidural experience nausea or vomiting compared with 1 percent of women who don't have epidurals.[38, 42, 65] (See also "Taking a Deeper Dive.")

   • **Itching.** A minimum of 3 percent of women who have an epidural experience itching compared with less than 1 percent of women who don't have epidurals.[3, 47]

   • **Postpartum urinary retention (inability to urinate or to completely empty the bladder after the birth).** A minimum of 18 percent of women who have an epidural experience postpartum urinary retention compared with a maximum of less than 1 percent of women who don't have epidurals.[3]

   • **Post-dural-puncture headache, also called "spinal headache."** In about 1 percent of epidural procedures,[32] the needle accidentally pierces a hole in the dural membrane. Roughly 80 percent of women to whom this happens develop a severe headache after the birth.[4, 51, 56, 71] (See also "Taking a Deeper Dive.")

   • **Recurrent headache or backache as a long-term consequence of dural puncture.** About 60 percent of women who experience dural puncture go on to experience recurrent headache and about 50 percent experience chronic backache.[4, 51, 56, 71] This can continue for as long as eighteen months after the birth. Eighteen months is the longest studies to date have followed up, which means we don't know how long headaches or backaches might continue. Women who had accidental dural puncture were also more likely than women who had uneventful epidurals to report that headaches or backaches in the months after birth were severe.[4, 51, 71] Since 1 percent of women who have an epidural experience dural puncture and 60 percent of women who have a dural puncture experience recurrent headache, then multiplying 1 percent by 60 percent tells us that 0.6 percent, or 6 per 1000 women who have an epidural, will experience post-dural-puncture-related recurrent headache. Similarly, since 50 percent of women who have a dural puncture experience chronic backache, then multiplying 1 percent by 50 percent tells us that 0.5 percent, or 5 per 1000 women who have an epidural, will experience post-dural-puncture-related chronic backache. (See also "Taking a Deeper Dive.")

6. **Epidurals can cause low blood pressure (*hypotension*), which can lead to fetal distress.** Despite receiving IV fluid to bolster blood volume and avert this complication, 30 to 40 percent of women who have an epidural will experience hypotension.[32] Maternal hypotension can lead to fetal distress, and, in fact, having an epidural may slightly increase the risk of having a cesarean for fetal distress (3 percent versus 2 percent).[3]

7. **On rare occasions, epidurals cause life-threatening or severe complications.** Life-threatening complications include *high blockade* (the anesthetic migrates upward, paralyzing breathing muscles and the heart) and systemic toxic reaction to the anesthetic. Rates of occurrence are reported at 2 to 7 per 10,000 women having epidurals.[52, 60] Epidurals can also damage nerves serving the legs either directly during administration or through bleeding accumulating (*hematoma*) in the epidural space, with rates reported at 1 in 2600 to 1 in 220,000 women who have an epidural.[32] The injury can result in long-term or even

permanent weakness. No data were reported for how often long-term or permanent weakness results from nerve injury.

◊ **8. Epidurals can cause maternal fever and therefore its adverse effects.** Women who have an epidural are more likely to run fevers in labor (22 percent versus virtually no women who don't have an epidural).[33] (See also "Taking a Deeper Dive.") Fevers can lead to:

- **A possible increased likelihood of instrumental (vacuum extraction or forceps) delivery or cesarean surgery.** For information on the adverse effects of instrumental delivery, see "Instrumental (vacuum extraction or forceps) vaginal delivery" under "9. Epidurals can impede labor …" in "Taking a Deeper Dive." As for cesareans, the list of the adverse effects of cesareans is so long that it would take up too much space to list them all. Suffice it to say that a cesarean is major surgery with all that entails in terms of pain, risk, and recovery, and that its harms include increased risks to mother and baby in future pregnancies.

- **Maternal antibiotic treatment.** Women who have an epidural are more likely to be given antibiotics compared with women who don't (14 percent versus 9 percent).[33] Antibiotics pass into breast milk, which is problematic because they kill the good bacteria as well as the bad and the resultant vacuum creates an opportunity for yeast to grow.[73] Yeast infections of the nipples and baby's mouth (*thrush*) make breastfeeding painful for both parties.

- **Increased probability of neurologic symptoms such as seizure in the newborn.** The difference is small—2 more newborns per 1000 mothers who ran fevers—but babies born to mothers who ran fevers in labor are more likely to experience neurologic symptoms such as seizure than babies of mothers whose temperature remained normal.[49]

◊ **9. Epidurals can impede labor, which can lead to interventions to address that problem, all of which have potential adverse effects.** Epidurals tend to lengthen both the dilation and pushing phases of labor, and they increase the probability of the baby persisting in an unfavorable position for descending through the pelvis (*persistent occiput posterior*). (See also "The Deeper Dive.") Slow or non-progressing labor leads to:

- **IV oxytocin to strengthen contractions.** It's hard to get a handle on additional use of IV oxytocin because it's so commonly used in labors regardless of circumstances, including in women progressing normally.[12] One study, though, found that 74 percent of first-time mothers who had epidurals had oxytocin compared with 20 percent of those who didn't.[62] (See also "Taking a Deeper Dive.")

- **Instrumental vaginal delivery.** A minimum of 4 more per 100 first-time mothers who have an epidural will have an instrumental vaginal delivery compared with first-time mothers who don't have an epidural (19 percent versus 15 percent),[3] but the actual difference is probably higher. Three other studies report a range of 9 to 19 more first-time mothers per 100 who have an epidural also having an instrumental delivery (21 percent versus 12 percent; 15 percent versus 5 percent; 27 percent versus 8 percent).[24, 50, 62] (See also "Taking a Deeper Dive.")

- **Arguably, cesarean surgery.** Majority obstetric opinion holds that research has shown that epidurals don't increase the likelihood of cesarean surgery. I think equally compelling studies conclude that they do, and there are weaknesses in the studies concluding that they don't. Two of the studies I find compelling looked at first-time mothers at low risk for cesarean and found, respectively, that 6 and 10 more per 100 who had an epidural had a cesarean (8 percent versus 2 percent; 15 percent versus 5 percent).[24, 50] A third study of a mixed population of low-risk first-time mothers and women with prior births found that 12 more per 100 women who had an epidural would have a cesarean compared with women who didn't (20 percent versus 8 percent).[6] (See also "Taking a Deeper Dive.")

All that said, the care provider you choose can affect your chances of cesarean surgery more than any other factor. You can find more about this point in "Taking a Deeper Dive." Look under

"9. Epidurals can impede labor ..." for the subheading "Arguably, cesarean surgery."

◊ **10. Having an epidural increases the probability of postpartum hemorrhage.** Women birthing vaginally who experienced a postpartum hemorrhage (defined as losing 1000 mL [2 pints] of blood or more after the birth or requiring a transfusion) were more likely to have had an epidural (30 percent versus 24 percent).[46] That said, only 5 percent of women in the population that produced this data had a postpartum hemorrhage, so this suggests the effect of an epidural will be quite small. (See also "Taking a Deeper Dive.")

◊ **11. Epidurals interfere with the production of hormones that regulate breastfeeding, mediate the woman's experience of labor, and influence her maternal feelings toward the baby.**[18, 35, 63] (See also "Taking a Deeper Dive.")

◊ **12. Epidurals lead to more babies being born in poor condition.** Babies of mothers who have epidurals are more likely to have 5-minute Apgar scores less than 7 (20 versus 11 per 1000, or 9 more babies per 1000 whose mothers had epidurals) and to have 5-minute Apgar scores less than 4 (3 versus 2 per 1000, or 1 more baby per 1000).[57] (The Apgar score evaluates the baby's condition at set intervals after birth on a scale of 1 to 10 with 10 being the highest score and 1 the lowest.) Babies of mothers who have epidurals are also more likely to be admitted to a *neonatal* (newborn) intensive-care nursery (7 versus 4 per 1000, or 3 more babies per 1000 whose mothers have epidurals).[57] (See also "Taking a Deeper Dive.")

◊ **13. Epidurals probably have adverse effects on breastfeeding.** Epidurals are associated with earlier breastfeeding discontinuation, more reports of problems with milk supply, and more formula supplementation.[23, 31, 68, 70] (See also "Taking a Deeper Dive.")

A FLY IN THE OINTMENT:
ANOTHER FACTOR IN PLAY

Now that I've listed the adverse effects of epidurals, you may be thinking about making an epidural "Plan B" to avoid them. Unfortunately, if you are getting usual labor management from a typical obstetrician, that probably won't work. This is because usual labor management includes frequent use of induction of labor, preset time limits for making progress in labor, routine use of fetal monitoring, IVs, no oral intake, rupturing membranes, and a low threshold for deciding to use cesarean or instrumental vaginal delivery. You might avoid some adverse effects—fever, for example—but you will likely have roughly the same probability of having continuous fetal monitoring, IV fluids, IV oxytocin, and an instrumental vaginal delivery or cesarean delivery as if you'd had an epidural. That means you will have the same probability of experiencing their adverse effects.

As for why typical obstetric management overuses medical interventions, the reasons include:

#1 Beliefs in the harmlessness of cesarean surgery.

I always tell people that an easy C-section is better than a hard vaginal delivery.[45]

#2 Economic incentives.

NPR's Shankar Vedantam provides a simple answer: "Obstetricians perform more cesarean sections when there are financial incentives to do so," citing a study conducted by the National Bureau of Economic Research (NBER), which analyzed the links between "economic incentives and medical decision-making during childbirth."[72]

#3 Defensive medicine.

The minute you see a deceleration on the heart monitor, you say maybe it's fetal distress, better to do a cesarean … . A lot of that is driven by fear of liability.[14]

#4 Convenience.

"Scheduling an induction can make everyone's life easier," [Dr. Leveno] said … . "I am not capable of constantly doing my best work in the middle of the night."[69]

Finally, if you are wondering whether practitioners resort to high use of medical intervention because it has been shown to improve outcomes, numerous studies have concluded that it does not. Not to worry, though, I'll be covering strategies for countering this problem in the "Take-Away" chapter.

IN SUMMARY

- Epidural analgesia has one unrivaled advantage: it is the only strategy capable of completely relieving pain.

- Obtaining that benefit, however, involves many offsetting disadvantages.

- Choosing to avoid an epidural may not garner all the potential benefits of that choice. This is because as I discussed in "A Fly in the Ointment," typical obstetric management involves frequent or routine use of practices that are necessary for epidurals but not necessary for most women.

TAKING A DEEPER DIVE
CAUTION: DENSE INFORMATION ZONE AHEAD

This section is supplemental material. It isn't intended to be read from beginning to end—unless you're looking for a sleep aid, in which case it should do the job, has no side effects, and isn't habit forming.

Jokes aside, I've included it as a cross-check to help you decide who to believe when you hear information contradictory to what I've told you or in case you want to know more about the "whys" of epidurals. I've put it here rather than in the main body of the chapter to separate it from the essential knowledge you need to decide whether you want to plan an epidural.

Accordingly, this section will give you the details of my analysis of the research and my reasoning processes so you have what you need to form your own opinion. It will also lay out problems with the research disregarded by mainstream obstetric practitioners, which leads them to portray an overly rosy picture of epidurals. And finally, if you're curious about *why* epidurals cause the problems they cause, I've got some explanations for you.

Before you look at the specifics of what's covered in this section, though, please read "Problems with the Research." It will help you understand my research analysis.

PROBLEMS WITH THE RESEARCH

The "Epidural Disadvantages" section gives you numbers so you know how likely you are to experience a particular adverse effect, but as I cautioned earlier, those numbers aren't as straightforward as you would think because there are problems with the research that produced them. Here are those problems:

Problem #1

To begin with, some of the data comes from *randomized controlled trials* (studies in which participants are randomly assigned, i.e., by chance, to one form of treatment or another and outcomes are reported according to assignment group) or from *systematic reviews* of randomized controlled trials (analyses of data pooled from multiple trials).

A strength of this study design is that it eliminates the possibility that differences in outcomes are attributable to differences in the participants rather than attributable to the intervention being studied. For example, if more women who have epidurals have cesareans, is that because epidurals lead to cesareans or because women having difficult labors—who are therefore more prone to having cesareans—are also more likely to want epidurals? Which is cause and which is effect?

A randomized controlled trial can answer that question, but there's a problem with the epidural trials: this study design only works when participants almost all get the treatment to which they were assigned. In the epidural trials, however, substantial percentages of trial participants assigned to avoid an epidural had one anyway. This crossover diminishes the difference between groups and makes it more difficult to determine the actual effect of an epidural. Large amounts of crossover could lead either to falsely finding no difference between women having versus not having an epidural or to finding a difference that is smaller than the actual difference. When I'm reporting results from randomized controlled trials, I'll use *assigned* and *planned* to alert you to this caveat.

Problem #2

A second problem is that the standard epidural anesthetic mixture includes an opioid, and all but a few women in the "avoid epidural" group would have had opioids too. This is because opioids via IV or injections were the alternative pain-management strategy to epidurals. That means trials are comparing women having opioids via an epidural with women having opioids intravenously or via injection, not to women having no opioids. (Some doctors and nurses believe that epidural medications don't get into the maternal bloodstream or cross the placenta into the baby's circulation, but we've known for decades that they do.[25, 44, 58]) Results, therefore, will underestimate the actual effect of epidurals for any opioid-related adverse effect.

For example, opioids are notorious for resulting in drowsy babies who are slow to start breathing. A systematic review of randomized controlled trials reported that fewer babies whose mothers were in the planned epidural group had low blood pH—an indicator of low oxygen—at birth or needed naloxone (Narcan), which counteracts opioid-induced respiratory depression.[3] All that tells us is that epidurals look good compared with women who receive injected or IV opioids. It tells us nothing about how epidurals would compare with undrugged women.

Problem #3

A third problem is that epidurals require continuous monitoring, IV fluids, and restriction to bed and often require use of IV oxytocin. These procedures and restrictions are not usually needed for women who don't have epidurals, but typical medical management of labor often includes them anyway. Therefore, studies are comparing women with epidurals with women who aren't having epidurals but who are nonetheless undergoing the same procedures and restrictions, all of which have potential adverse effects. For example, continuous fetal monitoring increases the likelihood of cesarean delivery.[1] This masks the actual effect of epidurals.

Problem #4

Finally, studies often lump together first-time mothers with women who have had previous births. First-time mothers are much more susceptible to factors that impede progress, so including women with prior births can make it appear that epidurals are not problematic or are less problematic for first-time mothers than they really are.

To repeat what I said above, *all of this is to say that when you look at the numbers in trials of planned epidural versus planned avoidance of epidural, you are looking at the best-case scenario for epidurals.*

EPIDURALS REVISITED

As promised, I'll now revisit the list of items from this chapter's main discussion for which I have additional information. The numbers here match up to the numbers in the main section, but because I've not included additional information for every item, some numbers are skipped here. Hopefully, my system will help you jump quickly to what interests you.

Happy exploring!

◊ 2. **Epidurals convert birth into a medical process controlled by medical staff.**

In this discussion, I'll step away from my neutral stance of presenting the facts as I understand them and address the assumptions that underlie the dominant model of care. I'm taking this step because I want to present another model that is based on different assumptions. You can't decide whether it attracts you if you don't know it exists. And because the dominant model is so … well … *dominant*, you may never learn about it if I don't tell you about it here.

As I said above, the dominant medical model conceptualizes childbirth as a solely physical process to be managed by medical professionals. The goal is to deliver a baby as efficiently and painlessly as possible, and the labor experience, other than controlling pain, has little importance in this model. (See also "The Pain Relief/Satisfaction Paradox" in Chapter 5.) In contrast, the physiologic care model centers on the woman as birth giver, and care takes into account the emotional, psychological, and spiritual aspects of childbirth. This model permits conceptualizing birth as a rite of passage, that is, a transformational event for which the pregnant woman is prepared and guided by people whose knowledge and wisdom she trusts. Within this model, labor can become a peak experience that challenges a woman to her core, and from which she emerges a changed person with a deepened knowledge of who she is and what she is capable of.

Not everyone wants this kind of experience, of course, in the same way that not everyone wants to spend a week in the woods with only the bare necessities or run a marathon or take up skydiving, and fortunately, when it comes to birth, epidural analgesia has made it a choice for those who don't. If it does appeal to you, though, you need to know that planning an epidural eliminates this possibility. Let me explain why.

By its nature, a rite of passage puts you at the center. It's about you struggling, striving, accessing your resources (both inner and outer), overcoming your fears, and finding your strength. It's about the love, support, and assistance of those who are with you.

By contrast, once you have an epidural, the medical team is in charge, and you become "done to" rather than "doing." You feel little or nothing. You are detached from your body from the waist down. You can check your phone or sleep or chat as you please. You might be able to move your legs a bit, but you are confined to bed and connected to tubes, wires, and machines. You no longer have an active role to play. Hospital staff will use the incoming data gathered from the monitoring equipment to manage your labor and your and your baby's physical status.

This loss of agency and sensation has consequences. It's like being chauffeured to a campsite where the tent has been pitched for you and a staff prepares your meals, or driving the marathon route, or watching a film made by a skydiver wearing a helmet cam. You don't need to dig deep into the skills and knowledge you acquired in preparation for your wilderness adventure; you don't need people cheering you on from the sides of the road and handing you water bottles as you pass by; you don't need to conquer the terror of stepping out of an airplane into open air. You end up with a baby in your arms at the end, but it's not the same experience getting there. It can't be.

At this point, you might be intrigued. If you are, your next thought may be: "But what if I can't hack it, and I end up with an epidural anyway? Then I'll feel awful about myself. Wouldn't it be better not to take that risk?"

To this concern I answer, first, that there are ways to maximize your odds. I cover them in the "Take-Away" chapter. And second, it's all in the framing. Deciding in labor that an epidural has become your best option isn't a failure any more than tripping during a marathon and not being able to finish the race. Disappointing, yes, but not a failure.

OK, I hope I've given you what you need to decide whether you want to go further down this track. Back to our regularly scheduled programming.

◊ 5. **Epidurals can have unpleasant side effects.**

These include:

- **Nausea or vomiting.** This and itching, the next one on the list, are due to the opioid component of the epidural anesthetic mixture. According to a systematic review, 10 percent of women assigned to the planned epidural group experienced nausea or vomiting, compared with 15 percent of women assigned to the planned avoidance of an epidural group.[3]

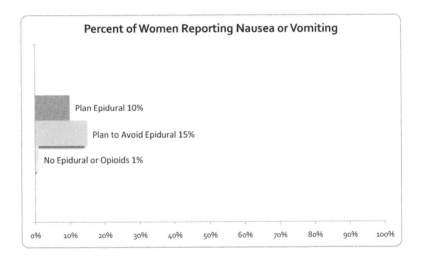

In other words, 5 fewer women per 100 planning an epidural experienced nausea or vomiting. Going by this review, women assigned to planned epidurals do better in this regard than women assigned to avoid an epidural.

This, though, is an example of problem #2 on my "Problems with the Research" list because almost all women assigned to avoid an epidural would have gone on to have IV or injected opioid medication for their pain. This means the trial compared women who had opioids via one route with women who had opioids via another route, and, if the women opted for an epidural, possibly opioids from both routes. However, I have data from trials of other pain-relief methods that reported nausea and vomiting rates in women who didn't have opioids at all.[38, 42, 65] In these women, only 1 percent experienced nausea or vomiting. So, instead of 10 percent versus 15 percent, we now have 10 percent versus 1 percent. In other words, we now have 9 *more* women per 100 in the epidural group experiencing nausea or vomiting compared with women who had neither an epidural nor opioids.

- **Post-dural-puncture headache, also called "spinal headache."** Because the epidural needle needs to be big enough to pass a catheter through it, the resultant hole when the dural membrane is accidentally punctured can leak enough fluid to cause a drop in cerebrospinal fluid pressure. Doctors aren't sure why the loss of pressure causes excruciating headaches.[71] They think it may have something to do with the resultant pull on pain-sensitive tissues.

- **Recurrent headache or backache as a long-term consequence of dural puncture.** Doctors have long thought that recovery from post-dural-puncture headache was the end of the problem, but accumulating research suggests that this is not the case and, as we saw in the main section, that women experiencing accidental dural puncture in labor may go on to develop recurrent headache and chronic backache extending out many months after the birth. Researchers have a couple of theories on why this might happen. One is that the puncture doesn't heal completely and continues to leak, causing ongoing headache (or backache), and the other is that similar to other chronic headache syndromes, the tissues become sensitized and prone to recurring symptoms.[71]

◊ **8. Epidurals can cause maternal fever and therefore its adverse effects.**

One explanation for more fevers could be that epidurals can lengthen labor, which might allow more time for infection to develop. However, we know that epidurals are the culprit, not infection developing over the course of a longer labor, because the likelihood of fever increases with *epidural* duration but not with *labor* duration. In the absence of an epidural, fever rates remain low regardless of labor duration.[41]

◊ **9. Epidurals can impede labor, which can lead to interventions to address that problem, all of which have potential adverse effects.**

Epidurals tend to lengthen both the dilation and pushing phases of labor, and they increase the probability of the baby persisting in an unfavorable position for descending through the pelvis (*persistent occiput posterior*).

Before we get to the consequences of this, though, let's talk about why epidurals do this. The problem is that numbing nerves, the intended effect of epidurals, also has unintended effects that interfere with labor progress.

For one thing, numbing sensory nerves disrupts the feedback mechanism that orchestrates labor progress. Here's how the feedback mechanism works: sensory nerves transmit sensation and stretching to the brain, which responds by secreting various hormones and hormone-like substances, whose job it is, among other things, to intensify contractions, trigger the waves of urge to bear down, and supply laboring women with energy and strength.[2, 8, 13, 18, 55, 67]

For another, the anesthetic numbs motor nerves, not just sensory nerves, which prevents mobility. We have evidence that being active in labor helps to promote labor progress.[28, 39] One reason for this may be that upright postures put gravity in your favor. Upright, you have the weight of seven or more pounds of baby helping to dilate the cervix. Women who aren't numb often instinctively seek positions and activities that increase comfort. For example, they may walk, lean forward on a support and rock their pelvises, sway from foot to foot, etc. Not coincidentally, this helps position the baby favorably to enter and move through the pelvis.

Finally, numbing motor nerves may also contribute to persistent fetal malposition. What's the problem there, and how might that work?

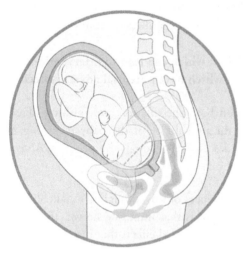

Figure 7: Occiput Posterior

As you can see in Figures 7 and 8, *occiput posterior* (OP) babies—that is, babies with the back of their heads (*occiput*) against the mother's back—present a broader diameter of their heads to the pelvic opening. This makes it more difficult for them to pass through the pelvis—think about trying to pull a tight turtleneck sweater over the flat top of your head instead of starting at the smaller crown at the back of your head—which results in much higher rates of instrumental vaginal and cesarean delivery.[20, 26, 40, 53]

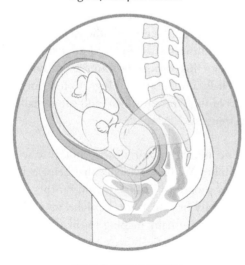

Figure 8: Occiput Anterior

Babies may face any which way in early labor,[40] but by the time the cervix is fully open and the baby has dropped into the pelvis, almost all babies have taken up the *occiput anterior position* (OA), that is, with the back of their head toward their mother's belly. The theory is that this happens because the muscle tone of the pelvic floor musculature guides the baby into the favorable OA position as the baby begins to descend into the opening in the pelvic bone.

Studies have found that epidurals are associated with increased probability of persistent OP baby.[11, 20, 26, 53] This makes sense if the above theory is correct. With an epidural, the pelvic floor would be relaxed and would not provide the proper resistance, making the swivel to OA less likely. It has been argued that the association between epidurals and persistent OP comes from women with OP babies experiencing longer, more painful labors and therefore being more likely to want an epidural. However, having an epidural remains an independent factor in studies that take into account other factors associated with persistent OP.[20, 64] Furthermore, pooled data from trials assigning women to planned epidural or planned avoidance of epidural groups also found more persistent OP babies in the planned epidural group (18 percent versus 13 percent).[3]

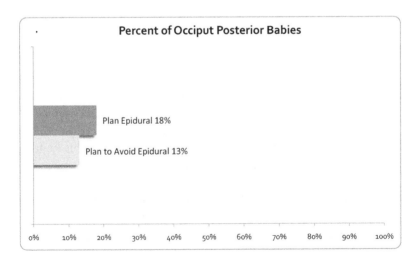

Finding an excess in random-assignment trials shoots down the theory that more difficult labors lead to epidurals. Indeed, the difference may be greater than it appears. Remember research problem #1: the actual difference between women who *have* an epidural and women who *don't* is probably greater than the difference found in trials comparing women *assigned* to planned epidurals versus *assigned* to avoid epidurals because substantial numbers of women assigned to avoid epidurals actually had one.

So, what are the consequences of this interference? Slow or non-progressing labor leads to:

- **IV oxytocin to augment contractions.** One adverse effect of IV oxytocin is *uterine hyperstimulation* (some combination of contractions that are too long, strong, or close together), which can lead to fetal distress. Another is postpartum hemorrhage.

  The systematic review I've been citing reported that roughly half (45 percent) of first-time mothers in both the planned epidural group and the group assigned to avoid epidurals had IV oxytocin to strengthen contractions.[3] This finding, however, is an example of both research problem #1— many women assigned to avoid an epidural actually had one, which diminishes differences between groups—and research problem #3—typical obstetric management involves use of labor interventions that most women don't need.

  For both those reasons, the systematic review isn't very helpful in determining the effect epidurals have on use of IV oxytocin. We have a study, though, that is. It included 5100 first-time mothers, nearly all (83 percent) of whom had epidurals.[62] This high a percentage tells us we're not just looking at a subset of women having difficult labors who might be more likely both to need IV oxytocin and to want an epidural. In this study, 74 percent of first-time mothers who had epidurals had oxytocin augmentation versus 20 percent of first-time mothers who didn't have epidurals.

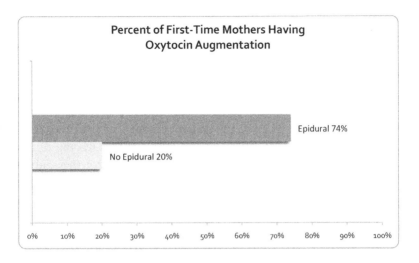

Percent of First-Time Mothers Having Oxytocin Augmentation

Epidural 74%

No Epidural 20%

0% 10% 20% 30% 40% 50% 60% 70% 80% 90% 100%

- **Instrumental (vacuum extraction or forceps) vaginal delivery.** Maternal adverse effects of instrumental vaginal delivery include increased use of *episiotomy* (snipping the vaginal opening to enlarge it for birth), more anal-sphincter tears, more cases of childbirth-related psychological trauma, and more cases of fecal incontinence later in life. Newborn adverse effects include increased stress and pain during delivery, which can interfere with bonding and breastfeeding, and more cases of *cephalohematoma* (a blood-filled swelling of the scalp). Rare severe newborn complications include *intracranial hemorrhage* (bleeding within the brain), seizure, facial-nerve injury, *brachial plexus injury* (injury to a nerve complex serving the shoulder and arm), and *subgaleal hemorrhage* (a life-threatening hemorrhage between the bottom layer of the scalp and the membrane covering the skull.)

The systematic review of trials of planned epidural versus planned epidural avoidance reported a modest increase in instrumental delivery (19 percent versus 15 percent, or 4 more first-time mothers per 100 allocated to planned epidural).[3] Again, though, this could be an example of research problem #1: substantial numbers of women assigned to avoid epidurals actually had one, which means the actual difference between groups could be greater.

Supporting that this is the case, studies comparing first-time mothers who had epidurals with first-time mothers who didn't report greater differences in instrumental delivery. One study reported that 15 percent versus 5 percent, or 10 more per 100 first-time mothers who had an epidural, had an instrumental delivery versus 5 percent who didn't.[62] Two other studies of first-time mothers made special efforts to rule out difficult labors leading to instrumental or cesarean delivery (more details on what they did under "cesarean delivery"). One reported that 21 percent versus 12 percent, or 9 more per 100, who had an epidural had an instrumental delivery,[24] and the other reported a difference of 27 percent versus 8 percent, or 19 more per 100, who had an epidural.[50]

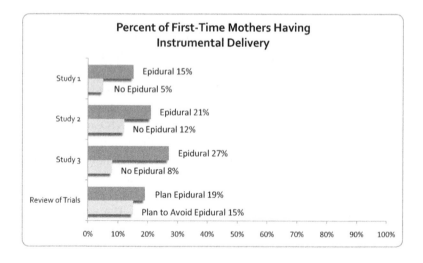

- **Arguably, cesarean surgery.** The list of cesarean adverse effects is so long that it would take up too much space to list them all here. Suffice it to say that a cesarean is major surgery with all that entails in terms of pain, risk, and recovery, and that its harms include increased risks to mother and baby in future pregnancies.

When it comes to the question of whether epidurals increase cesareans, I part company with majority opinion. If you ask almost any obstetrician and probably many midwives whether having an epidural increases the chances of cesarean, you will likely be told that this used to be a concern, but that research has shown it does not. That conclusion comes largely from the finding of the systematic review I've been citing in this chapter, which, indeed, reported nearly identical cesarean rates in women randomly assigned to planned epidural or to planned avoidance.[3] I disagree that this review is the final word. I think a strong case can be made that epidurals do increase cesareans—or at least they have the potential to do so. More on that hedge at the end of the cesarean surgery discussion.

To begin with, logic says that they should increase cesareans. As we have seen, epidurals interfere with labor progress, increase the probability of persistent OP baby, and increase the probability of fevers, all of which result in more cesarean deliveries. But if epidurals increase cesareans, why don't the random assignment trials show it? They don't, though. There's not a smidge of difference in cesarean rates even when you look just at trials in first-time mothers, who would be more vulnerable to any adverse effects of epidurals.

One group of dissenting researchers answers that question. To begin with, they point out that randomized controlled trials are generally conducted in academic centers in a hothouse environment of rules, protocols, and strict supervision. That means their results may not apply to the real-world conditions of the typical hospital and obstetrician.[6, 7] They also observe (as I have in this book) that analyzing outcomes according to assignment group can skew results when substantial proportions of participants receive the treatment of the other group. They then test whether this might have been the case with the trials in the systematic review. They apply a statistical analysis technique that compensates for the effect of crossover, and they find that, yes, epidural analgesia probably did, in fact, increase the probability of cesarean delivery.[7]

So far, we have reason to believe that data from randomized controlled trials may be misleading and that the finding that epidurals don't increase cesareans can't be taken as gospel. That casts doubt on the systematic review's conclusion but isn't conclusive. Do we have studies finding that epidurals increase cesareans?

If we turn to studies other than random assignment trials, we're back with the problem of how to tell whether an increase in cesareans is attributable to the epidural or whether it occurs because women with more difficult labors are more likely to want an epidural. Or are we?

I have three studies that addressed the problem of which came first: more difficult labor or the epidural. All three reported excess cesareans in women who had epidurals compared with those who didn't. Here's how the studies solved the chicken-versus-egg problem and their results:

The first of the three studies looked at first-time mothers at ultra-low risk of needing a cesarean.[24] To rule out that difficult labor led to the epidural, not vice versa, investigators used a diagnosis of prolonged labor as an indicator of difficult labor. They then applied a statistical technique that adjusted the results according to whether women had been given this diagnosis. After the adjustment, they found that more ultra-low-risk first-time mothers who had an epidural had a cesarean (8 percent versus 2 percent).

The other two studies used an analytic strategy called *propensity score matching*, a technique that like random assignment, addresses the possibility that the adverse outcome is related to the reason for the treatment, not the treatment itself. It works like this: using a long list of factors, investigators construct a propensity score using factors associated with how likely each study participant would be to have the treatment. In the case of these two studies, the treatment is an epidural, and the factors are such characteristics as induced labor, first birth, and birthweight. They then create matched pairs according to their scores in which one member of the pair has

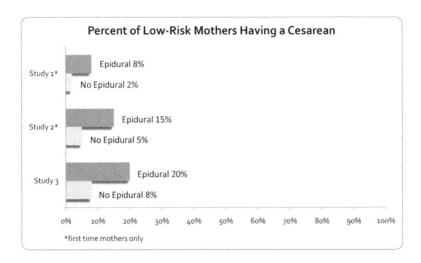

Percent of Low-Risk Mothers Having a Cesarean

Study 1*
Epidural 8%
No Epidural 2%

Study 2*
Epidural 15%
No Epidural 5%

Study 3
Epidural 20%
No Epidural 8%

0% 10% 20% 30% 40% 50% 60% 70% 80% 90% 100%

*first time mothers only

the treatment and the other doesn't, then compare results between the pairs. Using this technique, one study found that 15 percent of low-risk first-time mothers who had an epidural would have a cesarean versus 5 percent who didn't,[50] and the other study, which used a large database with detailed information to create nearly 53,000 matched pairs of women at low risk for cesarean, found 20 percent who had an epidural would have a cesarean versus 8 percent who didn't.[6]

However, as I said earlier, epidurals have the *potential* to increase cesareans but don't necessarily do so. This is because care-provider practice style overrides any effect of epidurals on a woman's probability of having a cesarean. Studies show that when care providers have low cesarean rates, epidurals don't increase the odds of cesarean.[10, 30, 34, 37, 61] This makes sense. You would expect that practitioners who have vaginal birth as a goal will have more patience and will manage labor and epidurals differently from those who are indifferent to whether labor ends in a cesarean. In other words, *epidurals slow labor, and they can lead to more cesareans, but whether they do also depends on care-provider philosophy and practices.*

◊ 10. **Having an epidural increases the probability of postpartum hemorrhage.**

Several factors may contribute to excessive blood loss with an epidural. To begin with, long hours on an IV oxytocin drip can tire out the uterine muscle so that the uterus doesn't contract down as it should after the placenta delivers. That tight contraction is needed to shut off maternal blood flowing from where the placenta detached. In addition, epidurals mean more *episiotomies* (a snip of the vaginal opening to enlarge it for birth) and more instrumental vaginal deliveries, both of which increase blood loss. Finally, my source for the increase only looked at women having vaginal birth. If, as some studies conclude, epidurals increase cesareans, then more cesareans would be an additional source of increased bleeding associated with epidurals because surgical delivery increases blood loss compared with vaginal birth.

◊ 11. **Epidurals interfere with the production of hormones that regulate breastfeeding, mediate the woman's experience of labor, and influence her maternal feelings toward the baby.**

I explained above about how numbing nerves short-circuits the feedback mechanism between sensory input and the hormones and hormone-like substances that orchestrate labor progress. But epidurals also interfere with the hormones that regulate breastfeeding, mediate how labor is experienced, and influence mothering feelings toward the baby.[18, 35, 63] Let's look closer at these hormones and what they do for you. Epidurals reduce secretion of:

- **Oxytocin.** Oxytocin, as you may already know, is responsible for uterine contractions, and surges of oxytocin produce the waves of the urge to push. Less well known are its effects on the brain. Oxytocin is produced by the pituitary gland, located deep within the brain, and is secreted into the cerebrospinal fluid as well as the bloodstream. Oxytocin has been called the "love" or "cuddle" hormone for its mental effects.[59] It is produced during sexual activity, in response to touch, and during breastfeeding, where it triggers the "let-down" reflex that releases milk from the mammary glands into the milk ducts. Oxytocin promotes feelings of well-being, trust, relaxation, and closeness to—in the case of new mothers—their partner and the baby. IV oxytocin, I should add, doesn't have these properties because it cannot cross the blood-brain barrier. One study found that women who had an epidural and IV oxytocin in labor still had deficient oxytocin levels two days after birth, which suggests that the combination may affect early breastfeeding.[35] More on that below.

- **Stress hormones (epinephrine, norepinephrine, cortisol).** The stress hormones provide not only energy to accomplish the birth, but also alertness afterward to greet and bond with the baby.

- **Beta-endorphin.** Beta-endorphin is the body's natural pain killer. You may have heard of it as the hormone that produces "runner's high." In birth, this translates to an exhilarated "top of the world," "I can do anything" feeling after the birth.

- **Prolactin.** Prolactin, sometimes called the "mothering" hormone, calms anxiety, mediates milk production, and fosters instincts to care for and protect the baby.

◊ **12. Epidurals lead to more babies being born in poor condition.**

Investigators found that the relationship between epidurals and poor condition at birth held for labors that began on their own as well as for induced labors and for spontaneous births as well as for instrumental vaginal deliveries. This suggests epidural analgesia has a direct effect on newborn condition at birth apart from increased use of IV oxytocin and instrumental delivery. This is plausible, given that epidurals increase length of labor, use of IV oxytocin (which makes contractions longer, stronger, and closer together), and instrumental and probably cesarean delivery.

◊ **13. Epidurals probably have adverse effects on breastfeeding.**

The research into epidural effects on breastfeeding is equivocal and difficult to interpret. Breastfeeding outcomes depend on many factors besides the use or non-use of epidural analgesia, and studies both finding and not finding an adverse relationship suffer from serious weaknesses.[27] Still, enough studies to raise concern took into account some of those factors and found that epidurals are associated with breastfeeding difficulties. The problems studies have found include earlier breastfeeding discontinuation, more reports of problems with milk supply, and more formula supplementation.[23, 31, 68, 70]

Additionally, what we know about epidurals makes a negative effect plausible. Let's look at some ways epidurals might adversely impact breastfeeding.

We've already seen that epidurals inhibit secretion of prolactin and oxytocin, hormones that regulate breastfeeding, and, in fact, a study reported that women having epidurals were more likely to experience a delay of more than 72 hours in the milk coming in (24 percent versus 11 percent).[43]

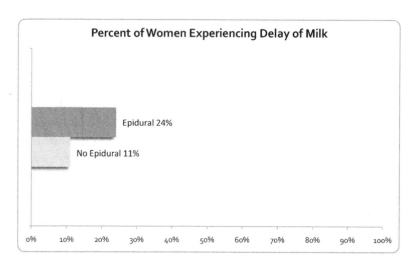

Several studies have found that epidurals disrupt instinctive newborn suckling behaviors. Babies of unmedicated mothers who are placed skin to skin on their mother's belly after birth will go through a predictable sequence of behaviors in which they propel themselves upward to their mother's breast, locate the nipple, explore it with mouth and hands, then latch on and begin suckling.[17] Babies of mothers who had epidurals are less likely to complete the sequence and achieve suckling.[16]

Fentanyl, the commonly used opioid component of the anesthetic mixture, may be the culprit in interfering with breastfeeding. Some studies have found that the more fentanyl the mother receives, the more likely to find an adverse effect on breastfeeding.[9, 16, 36]

Having IV oxytocin in labor may also have an adverse effect on newborn instinctive behavior,[17] and as we have seen, women having epidurals are more likely to require it.

Another problem stems from the large amounts of IV fluid that are given to try to prevent epidural-associated low blood pressure. That fluid can swell breast tissues, making it difficult for the baby to latch on properly in the first few days. To add to the problem, the baby's attempts to latch on can cause sore nipples. Excess fluids are also passed to the baby, artificially inflating the baby's birthweight by as much as several ounces.[19, 48] Breastfeeding adequacy is gauged by how long it takes to regain birthweight. Those extra few ounces could extend the time it takes, which could lead to thinking that milk supply is inadequate and prescribing formula supplementation unnecessarily. As beneficial as formula feeding may be when it is necessary, it can interfere with establishing milk supply and confuse the baby because the action of suckling at the breast and sucking a bottle nipple are different.

Finally, epidurals result in excess instrumental, and, as I have argued, cesarean delivery. The pain surgical delivery causes mothers, and instrumental delivery causes mothers and babies, is yet another obstacle to successful breastfeeding. Also, women having cesarean delivery are less likely to initiate breastfeeding in the first hour after birth, the so-called "golden hour" when mothers and their babies are primed to begin their relationship. This too interferes with establishing breastfeeding.

Chapter 3:
Combined
Spinal-Epidurals

A s the name suggests, combined spinal-epidurals (CSEs) are a subspe-
cies of epidurals in which the epidural is preceded by a related procedure called a "spinal." I decided to give the variant its own chapter, though,
because the epidural chapter was already complex enough without adding
another layer to the complexity.

I'm not actually sure CSEs are still being done, and because I don't know
whether they are or aren't and have no way of finding that out, I thought
I'd better cover them. However, instead of my usual practice for this book,
which is to give you the pros and cons of a labor-coping option as neutrally
as I can, I'm going to tell you why I think CSEs are a nonstarter as an
alternative to a straight-up epidural. Accordingly, I'm going to explain what
CSEs are and how they're done, poke holes in the rationales offered for

them, and make a data-supported case that they have no advantages and considerable disadvantages when compared with epidurals.

Here are three ways you could approach this chapter:

1. You can take my word for it and move on to another chapter.

2. You can cut to the chase and just read my summary at the end of this chapter.

3. You can read the chapter and decide whether you agree with my analysis.

WHAT IS A CSE?

A CSE is a two-stage procedure of which the second stage is an epidural. The first stage aka the spinal component is a single injection of either a) an opioid, b) a lower concentration of anesthetic than would be used for an epidural, or c) a mixture of both. The first-stage injection is delivered into the space inward of the epidural space. That is, the first stage is a *sub*dural injection—meaning beneath the dural membrane—instead of *epi*dural injection—meaning above the dural membrane. Unlike an epidural, in which a tiny, flexible tube (*catheter*) is left in the space to provide ongoing medication, the effect of the stage-one spinal injection only lasts an hour or two and can't be repeated. For this reason, the administration technique, which will be described in the next section, is designed to allow an easy conversion to stage two, the epidural.

WHAT'S INVOLVED IN ADMINISTERING A CSE?

The prep for the "spinal" stage of the procedure is the same as the prep for an epidural.[9] I'll summarize it for you here so that you don't have to turn back to the epidural chapter. As Figure 1 shows, the prep involves:

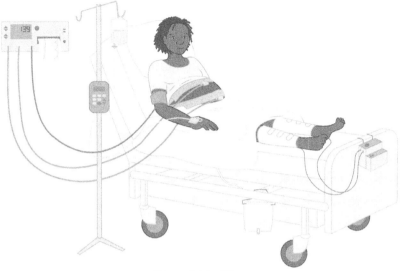

Figure 1: Epidural Prep

CSE PREP

- starting an IV,

- placing a blood-pressure cuff, usually automated so that it periodically inflates and deflates on its own,

- setting up continuous fetal monitoring, which involves putting two monitoring belts around the belly, one that uses ultrasound to pick up the baby's heartbeat and the other that has a sensor that picks up contractions,

- probably wrapping the legs in intermittent-compression cuffs that rhythmically inflate and deflate to help pump blood through them, and

- probably placing a urinary catheter to keep the bladder drained.

CSE ADMINISTRATION

After the prep is complete, next is the administration procedure. Figure 2 and Figure 3 illustrate this. To orient you, you're looking at a side view. The oblong shapes stacked vertically on the left depict the spinal vertebrae seen in cross section. The tube on the right is the dural membrane, which surrounds the spinal cord. The spinal cord—or more specifically at this level of the back, the bundle of nerves that emerges from the base of the spinal column—is shown as a darker column in the center of the tube.

As I said, CSEs are administered in a way that allows easy transition to an epidural when the spinal wears off. Here's how that's done:

The anesthesiologist (or nurse anesthetist) injects anesthetic to numb the skin. Then they slip a needle between the vertebrae of the lower back into the epidural space, which, as I said above, is the space just above the tough dural membrane that sheaths the spinal cord. Next, a much finer needle is passed through the bigger needle to pierce the dural membrane. Through it, the anesthesiologist injects the spinal dose into the space beneath the dura.[14] The

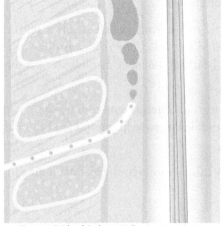

Figure 2: Epidural Needle Insertion

Figure 3: Epidural Catheter Delivering Anesthetic

fine needle that delivered the spinal injection is removed, and a tiny, flexible plastic tube (*catheter*) is threaded through the bigger needle into the epidural space. The larger needle is also withdrawn, and the catheter is left in place. The catheter is then taped to the back, ready for the epidural anesthetic when it is wanted.

Is There a Justification for CSEs?

The rationales for the spinal component have shifted over time, but none of them hold up to closer scrutiny.

The original justification was to overcome some of the disadvantages of the old-fashioned, high-dose epidural being used at the time, which caused profound numbness, completely paralyzed the legs, and significantly slowed labor. The spinal injection, it was thought, would provide pain relief while allowing some feeling and not compromising mobility. Having some sensation and unimpaired mobility would increase maternal satisfaction, and decreased paralysis would allow for more effective pushing, possibly reducing the need for instrumental delivery.[14]

This was muddy thinking, though, because, unlike an epidural, in which a catheter is inserted to provide ongoing medication, as I said, the spinal anesthetic injection only lasts an hour or two and can't be repeated. That limitation means that for most women, the spinal anesthetic injection would do no more than delay an epidural. So, at best, the spinal component would provide no more than one to two hours of additional mobile time.

In the 1990s, this limitation of CSEs started being touted as a feature. CSEs were deemed "walking epidurals"—something that would provide pain relief in early labor yet allow women to be up and around. The idea was that by the time the spinal anesthetic wore off, the labor would be more intense, and the woman would be ready to retire to bed with an epidural.

It seems unlikely, though, that many women would have walked with "walking epidurals." Even studies evaluating mobility with a CSE reported that less than half of the women with CSEs got out of bed. What's more, the definition of "mobile" in those studies could include sitting in a chair,[2, 14] which means an even smaller percentage who were designated as "mobile" actually walked. Hospital labor and delivery staff would have little motivation to promote mobility with a CSE. Getting women up and walking would add to the workload—women would need to be assessed, monitored, and possibly accompanied—and there would be concern about potential falls. Considering those disincentives, I'd imagine that few labor and delivery units in the 1990s and 2000s would have encouraged walking.

Today, no one seems to be talking about "walking epidurals." The modern prep for a CSE—involving as it does an IV, fetal monitoring belts, an automated blood-pressure cuff, and more—effectively tie a laboring woman to the bed.

Finally, the research literature talks about a spinal injection's faster onset compared with an epidural, but this amounts to an average six minutes faster from time of injection to time of effective analgesia.[14] Figure in the time it takes for the prep, and the time difference from request to relief—which is what would matter to the laboring woman—becomes meaningless.

That disposes of the justifications for CSEs. Let's see what the research has to say about their advantages—or lack thereof—compared with epidurals.

DO CSES HAVE ADVANTAGES COMPARED WITH EPIDURALS?

The research finds that compared with epidurals:[14]

- **CSEs don't increase mobility.** A *systematic review* (a study of studies on a particular topic) pooled data from trials that compared women assigned to have CSEs with women assigned to have a "light" epidural. The review found that women were no more likely to be mobile with the spinal component of a CSE than with a "light" epidural.[14]

- **CSEs don't decrease the cesarean rate.**[5, 14] In fact, they may possibly increase cesareans.[6] (See the "Disadvantages" section for more on this possibility.)

- **CSEs don't decrease the instrumental vaginal delivery rate.**[5, 14]

- **CSEs don't decrease rates of nausea or vomiting.**[14] They may even increase them.[5]

- **CSEs don't decrease likelihood of *post-dural-puncture headache* (a severe headache that develops after the birth).**[13]

DO CSES HAVE DISADVANTAGES COMPARED WITH EPIDURALS?

Not only do CSEs have no advantages over a straight-up epidural, some of the adverse effects they have in common with an epidural occur at higher rates. Compared with epidurals,

- **CSEs increase the likelihood of itching.** Fifty percent of women having a CSE versus 30 percent having an epidural experience itching.[14]

- **CSEs increase the likelihood of a worrisome episode of maternal low blood pressure (*hypotension*).** Six percent of women having a CSE versus 3 percent having an epidural experience an episode of low blood pressure severe enough to be given medication to treat it.[5]

- **CSEs increase the likelihood of an episode of worrisome slowing of the baby's heart rate during labor (*bradycardia*).** Ten percent of babies whose mothers have a CSE experience an episode of abnormally slow heart rate versus 4 percent of babies whose mothers had epidurals.[5, 6] If the slowdown is extreme and the heart rate doesn't recover within a short time, this could lead to a cesarean delivery, which raises the question: Do episodes of fetal bradycardia increase cesarean deliveries in women with CSEs?

Reviews pooling data from trials comparing CSEs with epidurals don't find more cesareans in women with CSEs.[5, 14] However, we have case reports and studies documenting rescue cesareans for this reason.[3, 4, 11, 12] Why, then, don't we see more cesareans in women with CSEs in the trials? I can think of a couple of reasons. First, it may be because women and babies in the trials were generally healthy and at full term. Their babies were therefore able to withstand the extra stress imposed by the medication. Second, it may also be because the excess number of babies experiencing bradycardia with a CSE is small. Only 6 more babies per 100 will experience bradycardia, and only some of those cases of bradycardia will result in cesarean delivery. A few extra cesareans would get lost in the noise of variation between groups that is due merely to chance. Interestingly, a couple of small trials looked specifically at the relationship between bradycardia and cesarean.[6] There weren't enough trial participants—less than two hundred in all—to come to a definitive conclusion, but it is suggestive that 9 percent of women in the CSE group versus 2 percent of women in the epidural group had a cesarean for this reason.[6]

And if that weren't enough, CSEs also have adverse effects not seen with epidurals. While both spinal and epidural administration involve opioids, injecting opioids into the cerebrospinal fluid bathing the spinal cord, as opposed to the epidural space, causes some unique complications:

- **Spinal opioid administration can cause difficulty swallowing.** Two women per 100 receiving spinal opioid will have such difficulty swallowing that they require treatment to reverse opioid effects.[1]

- **Spinal opioid administration can depress maternal breathing.** Six women per 1000 receiving spinal opioid will develop blood-oxygen levels low enough to require drug treatment to reverse opioid effects.[1] Respiratory depression may sometimes even devolve into respiratory arrest.[7, 8, 10]

IN SUMMARY

Combined spinal-epidurals offer no advantages over epidurals. Compared with epidurals, CSEs increase the likelihood of:

- itching,
- maternal low blood pressure requiring treatment, and
- worrisome slowing of the baby's heart rate.

The spinal component of CSEs also introduces adverse effects unique to them:

- difficulty swallowing serious enough to need treatment, and
- maternal respiratory depression concerning enough to need treatment.

Reviewers pooling data among trials of CSEs versus epidurals conclude:

There appears to be little basis for offering CSE over epidurals in labour.[14]

If a CSE is an option, you might want to pass. They increase the possibility of adverse effects with no counterbalancing benefits. My advice? If you want an epidural and you're offered a CSE, don't bother with an intermediary step. Go straight to an epidural.

Chapter 4:
Opioids

P rior to the development of epidurals and combined spinal-epidurals, opioids were the workhorse pain medication for labor. They are still available, but because epidurals completely relieve pain while opioids don't, epidurals have pretty much overtaken them.

Still, you might have reasons for considering an alternative pain medication to an epidural. You might not want to be numbed, or you may have a condition that contraindicates having an epidural. (If this describes you, see also Chapter 5, "Nitrous Oxide ['Laughing Gas']," for another non-epidural pain-relieving option.) Accordingly, as we did with epidurals and combined spinal-epidurals, let's look at how opioids are administered, how effectively they relieve pain, and their advantages and disadvantages.

WHAT'S INVOLVED IN ADMINISTERING OPIOIDS?

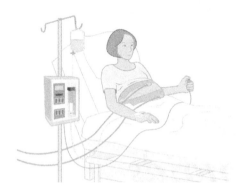

Figure 1: Patient-Controlled Analgesia

As you can see in Figures 1, 2, and 3, opioids can be administered via *patient-controlled analgesia* (PCA), or they can be injected into the IV line or into the hip muscle. With PCA, a pump permits you to self-administer a premeasured dose as you feel the need but has a lock-out mechanism to prevent overdosing.

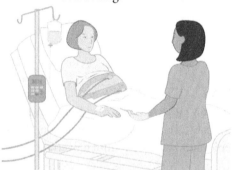

Figure 2: Injection via IV Catheter

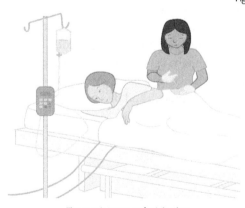

Figure 3: Intramuscular Injection

How Well Do Opioids Relieve Pain?

Opioids dull pain, but many women report continuing to experience moderate to severe pain.[15, 19] Surveys have found that while 62 percent of Canadian women and 75 percent of US women rated opioids as "very" or "somewhat" helpful, similar or higher percentages gave those same ratings to DIY strategies.[6, 13] These included hands-on techniques such as massage, deep-tub immersion in warm water, showers, position changes, application of heat or cold, mental strategies, music, and breathing techniques.

What Are the Advantages of Opioids?

Unlike epidurals:

- **Opioids don't substantially increase out-of-pocket birth costs.** The cost of an epidural may range as high as three thousand dollars even if you have insurance.[3, 5]

- **Opioids have a short delay between request and relief.** It can easily take an hour to get prepped for an epidural, have it administered, and have it reach full effect—and that's if the anesthesiologist is readily available. An opioid just requires a nurse to give an injection or set up an IV line.

- **Opioids don't affect mode of delivery.** An epidural increases the odds of an instrumental delivery, and while many obstetricians don't agree, a case can be made that epidurals can also increase cesarean delivery.

- **Opioids don't cause severe or life-threatening complications.** Life-threatening events are rare with an epidural, but they do happen. Opioids have adverse effects, but not ones that fall into this category.

DIY strategies, however, have these same advantages, and, as we just saw, they are about as effective as opioids at reducing pain.

WHAT ARE THE DISADVANTAGES OF OPIOIDS?

Unlike epidurals, the adverse effects of opioids are well established and undisputed. The difficulty comes in determining how likely you are to experience them because the data leave a lot to be desired. The studies we have are mostly trials with few participants that compare various opioid medications, each of which may function differently, and which were administered in various ways and according to various protocols—all of which could affect results too. And if that weren't enough, adverse effects were measured in different ways by different researchers. Not surprisingly, this has resulted in occurrence rates that are all over the map. Hopefully, though, I can still give you something useful to help guide your decision.

There is a winner among the opioids: remifentanil. Remifentanil, a newer opioid, is highly potent but is metabolized in less than two minutes, whereas other opioids take hours to metabolize. These unique characteristics enable it to be used via PCA to manage pain contraction by contraction.[19] Because it is so potent, it beats other opioids in relieving pain (although it is not as effective as an epidural), and because it is metabolized so quickly, it is less likely to have adverse effects on the baby.[19]

I'll go into details below on how remifentanil compares with other opioids. Unfortunately, though, you don't get to pick your opioid. You get what's on tap at your hospital. However, if remifentanil is available, that might enter into your decision as to whether you want an opioid.

Let's start with opioids' adverse effects in women:

- **Opioids can cause nausea and, less commonly, vomiting.** When I pooled results from studies of the same opioid administered in the same way, the percentages of women experiencing nausea ranged from 8 to 40 percent, depending on drug and method of administration.[15, 19] However, several results fell in the 17 to 23 percent range, including remifentanil, so I would say that 20 percent is a reasonable ballpark figure. This compares with a 9 percent rate with an epidural,[19] or about half the percentage of women having injected or IV opioids.

Epidurals, though, are the wrong comparison group because as we saw in the epidural chapter, the epidural anesthetic mixture includes an opioid, which means women having epidurals are getting opioids too, just by a different route. The right comparison group is women not having opioids at all. In these women, the nausea rate is a mere 1 percent.[8, 9, 15] Put another way, roughly 19 more women per 100 having injected or IV opioids will experience nausea compared with women not having opioids.

- **Opioids can cause itching.** Among women having an opioid, 3 to 6 percent will experience itching. Rates fall in the same range with an epidural,[1, 19] undoubtedly because they contain opioids too. This compares with less than 1 percent in women not having opioids.[1, 11]

- **Opioids have a sedative effect.** Drowsiness might seem to be a feature, not a bug, but it has drawbacks. It can make it more difficult for women to cope with contractions while making it appear that they are now comfortable and not in need of help from labor companions.[16] Sedation can also have consequences after the birth. Sometimes called the "golden hour," the first hour or so after birth is a unique period when mother and baby are hormonally primed to be alert and aware and ready to engage with each other and to get breastfeeding off to a good start. A sedated mother loses this opportunity.

- **Opioids can interfere with normal hormone secretion.**[4] Because opioids take time to clear the system, any effects they have may last for as long as a day or so after the birth. The research we have is scanty, but from what we know about how opioids work in the body and the effects observed in laboring women, the potential for interference and its adverse consequences are there. I've used "may" to indicate where the evidence is weakest.

  ◦ **Oxytocin.** Opioids inhibit oxytocin release, oxytocin being the hormone that causes uterine contractions and the waves of urge to push. Some data suggest that opioids slow labor progress,[4] although, as we saw above, opioids don't increase cesarean or instrumental delivery rates. However, oxytocin is also secreted into the brain, where it has mental effects, as well as the bloodstream.[14] It promotes feelings of love, well-being, and closeness, which would enhance affectionate feelings toward the baby. Oxytocin also triggers the let-down reflex that releases milk from the mammary glands.

- **Stress hormones (epinephrine, norepinephrine, cortisol).** Opioids reduce secretion of stress hormones, which sounds like a good thing except that these hormones provide energy during labor and ensure that women are alert and ready to greet and interact with their newborn.

- **Prolactin.** Opioids may inhibit prolactin release. Prolactin, sometimes called the "mothering" hormone, calms anxiety, mediates milk production, and fosters instincts to care for and protect the baby.

- **Beta-endorphin.** Because they reduce pain, opioids may also reduce beta-endorphin secretion. Beta-endorphins are responsible for "runner's high," that exhilarated "top of the world," "I can do anything" feeling after the birth.

Turning to adverse opioid effects on the baby:

- **Opioids can result in a baby who is slow to achieve normal respiration.** Opioids can sedate the unborn baby as well as the mother.[18] This can lead to a baby who is slow to breathe at birth, which can have several consequences:

  - **The baby may require resuscitation.** The percentage of babies requiring resuscitation ranges from 4 to 14 percent.[15] None of the studies of remifentanil reported incidence of resuscitation. I don't have a comparison number for babies who needed resuscitation whose mothers didn't have opioids. You would expect the number, though, to be no more than a few percent in healthy, full-term babies.

  - **The baby may require naloxone (Narcan) to reverse the opioid's effects.** For opioids other than remifentanil, the percentage of babies requiring naloxone ranges from 2 to 15 percent.[15, 19] Remifentanil via PCA is the standout here, with zero babies needing naloxone among five hundred women having remifentanil.[19] The need for naloxone administration is unique to the use of opioids.

◦ **The baby may require admission to an intensive-care nursery.** The percentage of admissions to neonatal intensive care ranged from 9 to 14 percent.[15] In most cases, admission will almost certainly be for a brief time for closer observation or extra care. I only have one study of 9 women reporting on this outcome with remifentanil. None of the babies required admission to an intensive-care nursery.[15] For comparison, in a large population of low-risk women beginning labor at a free-standing birth center or at home, 2 percent of babies required admission to newborn intensive care.[12]

Keep in mind that while respiratory effects can be reversed by injecting naloxone, having a sleepy baby and certainly the need for resuscitation would disrupt the "golden hour," the important "getting to know you" time right after birth as well as the opportunity to get breastfeeding off to a good start, which can affect breastfeeding success.

▪ **Opioids may reduce oxytocin secretion.**[4] Oxytocin is also secreted within the baby's brain and would likewise have a calming effect and foster feelings of well-being after the birth.

Finally …

▪ **Opioids can negatively impact breastfeeding.** Opioids inhibit effective suckling,[15] and because it may take days for the newborn's immature liver to clear opioids from their system,[15] the effect may persist beyond the early hours after birth. Also, opioid-exposed women are more likely to experience delay in the milk coming in,[10] which could be because sleepy babies who suck poorly don't stimulate the breast as well as they should. Some studies find that women having opioids are more likely to stop breastfeeding sooner,[17, 20] although other studies don't find a difference.[2, 7] It seems logical, though, that experiencing problems would lead to earlier breastfeeding cessation. Since remifentanil wears off so rapidly, it probably doesn't have the potential to affect breastfeeding as other opioids do, but I have no data on this point.

IN SUMMARY

Opioids do no better at relieving pain than DIY strategies, and unlike DIY strategies, they have adverse effects. Opioids:

- increase likelihood of maternal nausea,

- increase maternal and newborn sedation,

- increase occurrence of abnormal fetal heart rate,

- increase need for newborn resuscitation, and

- increase likelihood of problems with breastfeeding.

Although it still has the adverse effects common to all opioids, remifentanil stands out in that it does a better job of relieving pain and is less likely to have adverse effects on the baby.

Chapter 5:
Nitrous Oxide

I nhaling nitrous oxide (N2O), aka "laughing gas," was the other work-horse option for pain management along with opioids before epidurals came along. N2O fell out of favor in the US when epidurals entered the scene but not elsewhere in the world, where it has remained widely available. However, N2O has been making a comeback in the US in recent years,[11] and increasing numbers of hospitals offer it as an option.

N2O can't touch epidurals when it comes to relieving pain, but, as we'll see, it has other advantages, especially compared with opioids. As we've done in previous chapters, let's review what's involved in administering it, how well it relieves pain, and its advantages and disadvantages.

WHAT'S INVOLVED IN ADMINISTERING NITROUS OXIDE?

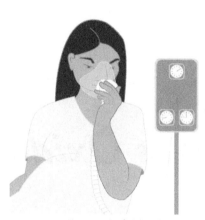

Figure: N2O Administration

Nitrous oxide, a scentless gas, is delivered in a 50:50 mixture with pure oxygen. When you feel the need, you trigger the flow by breathing in while holding the mask to your face. You breathe out into the mask as well, which enables the equipment to capture the gas and prevent it from escaping into the room.[10] Hand-holding the mask is a safety measure that prevents overdosing. Should you take in too much and become drowsy, your hand naturally falls away, and since N2O is rapidly metabolized, you quickly recover.

HOW WELL DOES NITROUS OXIDE RELIEVE PAIN?

Like opioids, N2O takes the edge off pain. Women rate N2O about on a par with opioids and, for that matter, about the same as DIY techniques such as mental strategies.[4, 8, 11]

N2O also has some psychological effects that can reduce pain *perception*, as opposed to relieving pain *sensation*. It can reduce anxiety,[8, 11] and as the name "laughing gas" implies, it can affect mood.[9] In other words, you still feel the pain, but you don't care.

THE PAIN RELIEF/SATISFACTION PARADOX

N2O presents us with a paradox: the same women who rate N2O as providing only moderate pain relief give N2O high satisfaction ratings.[11] How can this be? Isn't pain relief the most important consideration in coping with labor pain? Shouldn't there be a one-to-one correspondence between degree of pain relief and satisfaction? Anesthesiologists, most obstetricians and nurses, and not a few midwives would certainly think so.

It turns out, though, that "satisfaction" is a more complex concept than "hurting = bad"/ "not hurting = good." Satisfaction has to do with individual perspective, values, expectations, and context. For example, a study that explored this paradox with women found that women who were highly satisfied with N2O liked it even though it provided only moderate pain relief. They liked it because it put them in the driver's seat and furthered their goal of having an unmedicated birth.[11] They liked that it helped them feel less anxious and more relaxed and that its use distracted them from pain. They weren't looking to eradicate pain. They just wanted to reduce it to a tolerable level, and N2O fit that bill.

WHAT ARE THE ADVANTAGES OF NITROUS OXIDE?

Compared with epidurals and opioids, N2O offers a number of advantages:

- **N2O incurs minimal out-of-pocket cost.**[2] Epidurals can cost you hundreds, even thousands of dollars despite having insurance.[1, 3]

- **N2O is under your control.** You can decide in the moment when you want it and when you don't. As I explained in the text box, being in control is an aspect of satisfaction with the birth experience that can outweigh degree of pain relief for some women.

- **N2O provides immediate pain relief.** If you ask for the machine and to be shown how to use it when you arrive, it will be there when you want it, ready to use. That contrasts with preparing for and administering an epidural, which can easily take an hour from the time you make the request until the time that it starts to work—and that's if the anesthesiologist is readily available. And while the delay between requesting pain-relief medication and getting it will almost certainly be shorter with opioids than with epidurals, you are still dependent on waiting for the nurse to get to you, which may take longer than you would wish.

- **N2O doesn't interfere with mobility.** Epidurals prevent mobility because they numb motor nerves, and opioids may interfere because they can make you feel woozy. Being up and around can help labor progress and increases comfort.[5, 7]

- **N2O doesn't affect labor progress.** Epidurals, by contrast, can slow labor.

- **N2O doesn't appear to have adverse effects on the baby.** That's not true of opioids or epidurals.

- **N2O clears rapidly from the system.** N2O is gone from your system within a few minutes. If an epidural or opioid has an adverse effect, or you don't like how it makes you feel, you are stuck with it until it wears off, which will generally take an hour or more.

- **If N2O isn't cutting it, you can always step up to an epidural.** If you are on the fence about having an epidural, N2O provides an intermediate step between DIY strategies and an epidural.

WHAT ARE THE DISADVANTAGES OF NITROUS OXIDE?

N2O appears to have no serious adverse effects in mothers or babies. It occasionally has unpleasant side effects, however.

- **N2O can cause nausea and, less commonly, vomiting.** Six percent of women experience nausea.[4, 6, 8, 10] This compares with roughly 20 percent of women having injected or IV opioids.[12, 13]

- **N2O can cause dizziness.** Eight percent of women experience dizziness.[4, 6, 8, 10]

- **N2O use involves placing and removing a breathing mask.** This will not be possible where COVID-19 restrictions include wearing an air-filtration mask.

As I said above, an advantage of N2O is that its effects wear off rapidly when use is discontinued. On the other hand, though, only 1 percent of women laboring without analgesia experience nausea[6, 8, 12] and none will experience dizziness.

WHEN MIGHT NITROUS OXIDE BE A GOOD OPTION?

Here are some situations where I think N2O wins out over injected or IV opioid:

- **You plan to avoid an epidural, and you want more than DIY strategies in your toolbox.** As I said earlier, N2O can be a useful option for avoiding an epidural because it can be used as desired and mixed with DIY strategies.

- **You plan to delay an epidural until active labor, and you want a non-opioid analgesic in the meantime.** Why might you do this?

As we discussed in the epidural chapter, delaying an epidural until labor has kicked into high gear reduces the likelihood of developing an epidural-related fever and you or your baby experiencing the potential adverse consequences of that. It may also reduce your odds of cesarean, although whether the timing of epidural initiation affects the likelihood of cesarean is a matter of dispute. (See "Consider delaying an epidural until at least 5 cm dilation" in Chapter 7: "Your Take-Away.")

As we also discussed, you may wish to avoid an opioid because the standard epidural anesthetic mixture also includes an opioid, and the probability of you and your baby experiencing an adverse effect from opioids increases with accumulating dose.

- **You aren't a candidate for an epidural.** Some women have physical or health issues that rule out having an epidural.

- **You have to wait for your epidural, and you want something to help tide you over.** Having to wait can be very difficult once you have decided you want an epidural, and, as I noted above in this list, you may wish to avoid an IV or injected opioid. N2O gives you a non-opioid option that women rate as working equally well.

- **The epidural isn't working completely, and you're still in pain.** N2O may be a good choice for an add-on.

IN SUMMARY

- N2O offers some advantages over opioids and epidurals and is as effective at relieving pain as opioids.

- N2O's self-directed use and psychological effects make it highly satisfying to some women despite providing only modest to moderate pain relief.

- N2O can be useful for women who want to avoid an epidural and are finding DIY strategies insufficient.

- N2O can be useful for women planning an epidural but who wish to delay it until active labor; for women who must wait to receive their epidural; and for women whose epidural fails to relieve pain adequately.

- N2O can cause the same unpleasant side effects as opioids, but unlike opioids, N2O doesn't affect the baby adversely, and unpleasant effects should dissipate rapidly with discontinuing use.

Chapter 6:
DIY Strategies

L ast, but very much not least in our cavalcade of options for dealing with labor pain are DIY strategies. These are a variety of non-drug options that don't require medical staff to administer them.

Even if you are planning an epidural, I recommend that you go through this chapter. Its contents could be helpful under several circumstances: while you are still at home, if you wish to delay an epidural until active labor (see the epidural chapter for why you might want to do this), if you must wait until the anesthesiologist is available, or if you are one of the unlucky few for whom an epidural fails to work.

As usual, we'll start with what's involved, but before moving on to how well DIY strategies relieve pain and their advantages and disadvantages, I want to pause and talk about labor pain itself. I wrote a bit about the complexities of experiencing pain in the "Pain Relief/Satisfaction Paradox" in Chapter 5, "Nitrous Oxide ('Laughing Gas')," and I want to expand on what I wrote there in this chapter. I think it is important to do this because, as I wrote in the N2O chapter, the dominant societal view of labor pain is "hurting = bad"/ "not hurting = good." That black-and-white approach, however, oversimplifies a complex and varying intersection of context, perception, and interactions with others during the labor.

WHAT'S INVOLVED IN DIY STRATEGIES?

Unlike the pain-relief strategies in previous chapters, DIY Strategies are not a single method but cover a wide variety of possibilities. It's up to you to choose which ones you want to use and when you want to use them. There's a caveat, though: strategies that depend on a peaceful, private, quiet environment; or on supportive hospital policies; or on access to facilities such as showers, soaking tubs, or pools may be difficult or impossible to obtain in many hospitals.

The photos on the next few pages show you examples of some of the possibilities according to category. Photographs 1 and 2 illustrate social factors. These include supportive care from a birth partner, other loved ones, or both; and *doula care* (one-on-one care from a woman trained or experienced in labor support). Photographs 3 and 4 cover environmental factors such as privacy, dim lights, music, or aromatherapy. Photographs 5 and 6 offer examples of mental strategies, which encompass visualization, hypnosis, mindfulness, affirmations, using a visual focal point, patterned breathing, and prayer, while Photographs 7 and 8 show you physical strategies, a category that includes massage, acupressure, low-back counterpressure, reflexology, repetitive motion (swaying, rocking), and mobility (walking, positioning). Finally, we have Photographs 9 and 10, which demonstrate comfort measures such as warm-water immersion, showers, local application of heat, and local application of cold.

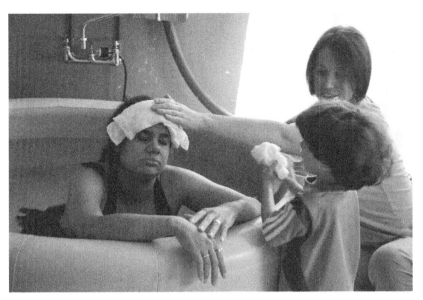

Photo 1: Social Factors

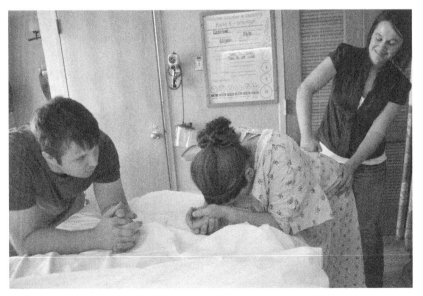

Photo 2: Social Factors

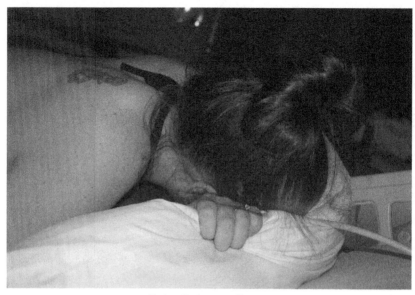

Photo 3: Environmental Factors

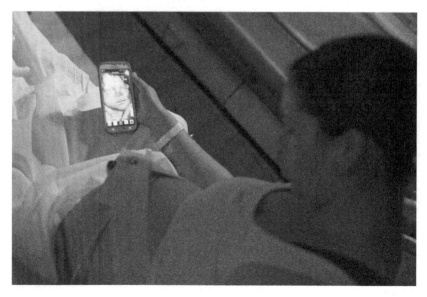

Photo 4: Environmental Factors

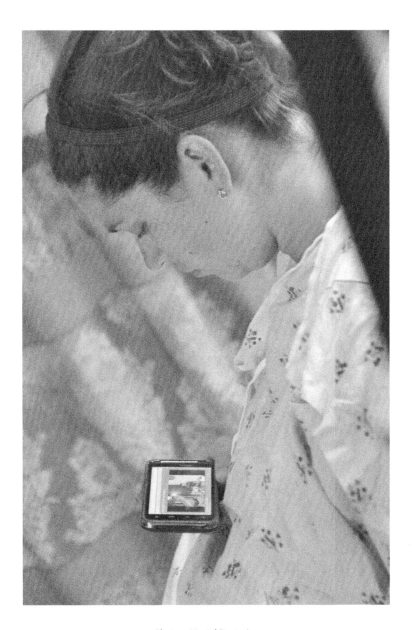

Photo 5: Mental Strategies

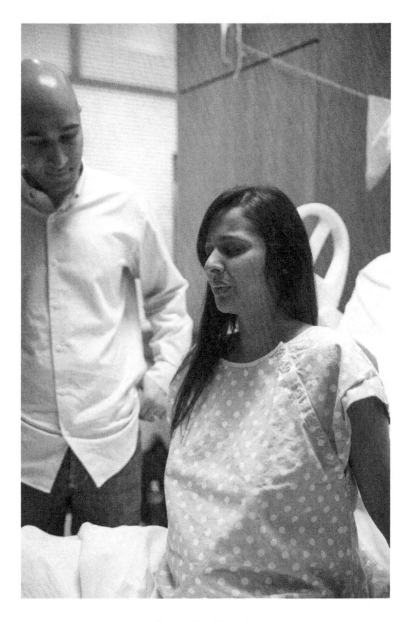

Photo 6: Mental Strategies

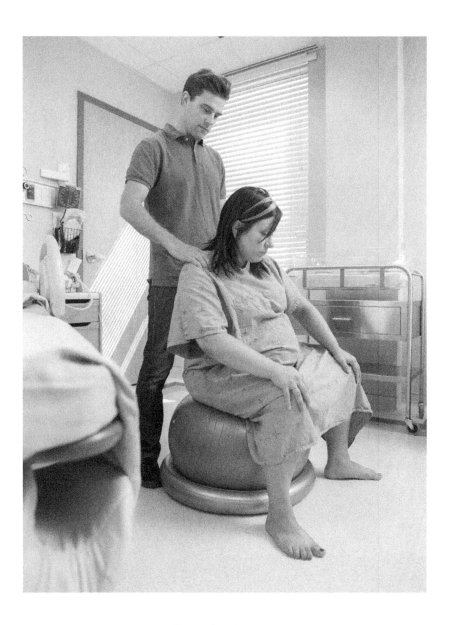

Photo 7: Physical Strategies

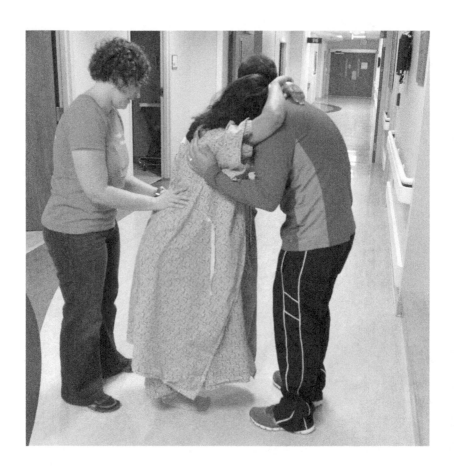

Photo 8: Physical Strategies

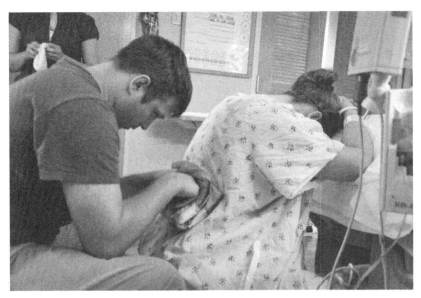

Photo 9: Comfort Measures

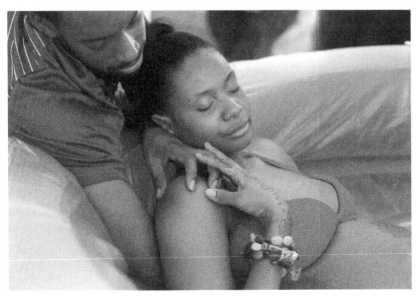

Photo 10: Comfort Measures

IS IT POSSIBLE TO HURT AND HAVE THAT BE OK?

As I said in the introduction, I'm now going to pause and talk about labor pain. The follow-on to the generally negative view of labor pain is that an epidural is the only way to cope with it. A popular argument in favor of epidurals goes something like this: either you labor comfortably with an epidural, or you try, probably unsuccessfully, to tough it out, and why would you want to suffer in the first place now that modern medicine has given you a choice?[14]

Before we go further, *I want to make it clear that I am in no way criticizing anyone who wants to avoid labor pain.* However, the reasoning behind this popular argument makes some underlying assumptions that bear closer examination. I want to surface and unpack them so that you have a fuller and more accurate picture, which will better enable you to decide where you stand.

> **Assumption #1: Labor pain has no redeeming value.** This assumption is made about labor pain but not about physical training or athletic contests, which are analogous instances in which effort involves pain. In those cases, many consider pain to be a normal and even desirable accompaniment to the process, as in the common phrase: "No pain, no gain." In other words, "labor pain has no redeeming value" is a personal judgment, not a fact.

> **Assumption #2: Labor pain is extreme to the point of being unbearable for the average person.** "Unbearable" is in the mind of the experiencer. The point at which it is reached varies from person to person. Moreover, as you can see in the table, labor pain differs physically and emotionally from pain arising from injury or illness in ways that can make a difference in how it is experienced.

How Does Labor Pain Differ from the Pain of Illness or Injury?

Labor Pain	Pain from Injury or Illness
Signifies something is happening as it should	Signifies something is wrong
Intensity builds gradually over time, which allows for adaptation	Is felt acutely from the time of onset
Ebbs and flows predictably, which allows preparing for it and anticipating relief	Is unpredictable in when it starts or stops or is felt strongly or less strongly
Is intermittent and brief, lasting only about a minute (back pain may be the exception)	Is usually continuous, and even cramping pain often has no pain-free interval
The degree of intensity is a sign of progress toward the goal	The degree of intensity is an indication of the severity of injury or illness
Experiencing intense pain is limited to hours at most	Experiencing intense pain may last for days or even longer

Assumption #3: The experience of labor pain is not modifiable. A study found that the experience of labor pain is shaped by two major factors.[29] One factor is the woman's perceptions. If she views her pain as positive, purposeful, and productive, she feels that she can cope without medication. If she views her pain as threatening, or if she experiences a mismatch between what she expected to be feeling and what she is experiencing, she feels that she needs medication. The other factor is the influence of those around her. If her caregivers, birth partner, or other labor companions are supportive, encouraging, and helpful, she will likely feel that she can cope without medication. If she feels unsupported, emotionally alone, and vulnerable, she will likely feel she needs medication.

The study also found that her interpretation of her pain is a dynamic process. For example, a woman may be coping well until she is examined and told she hasn't progressed as far as she thought, or a woman doubting her ability to continue without medication may have her confidence restored by a nurse's reassurances.

Assumption #4: Non-drug strategies do little or nothing to make labor pain manageable. This is the assumption behind the belief that only women with a high pain threshold will be able to get through labor without an epidural. As we'll see in the next section, that assumption isn't accurate.

To repeat the point I made in the N2O chapter, degree of pain relief and satisfaction with the birth experience don't necessarily correlate. Satisfaction with the birth experience depends on women:[1, 4, 6, 12–14, 19, 20, 22, 24, 26, 28]

- feeling emotionally and physically supported by their birth partner and other labor-support companions,

- feeling emotionally and physically supported by their caregivers and having them respect their preferences,

- being involved in decision-making,

- feeling in control over their environment and what happens to them, and

- feeling a sense of accomplishment and empowerment.

DIY strategies promote all of the above. So to answer the question posed in the title of this section, yes, it is certainly possible to hurt—even hurt a lot—and have it be OK, but it depends on several factors. The first is wanting this kind of birth; the second is planning and preparation for it; and the third is the luck of the draw because ultimately, you don't control how difficult or long the labor might be.

How Well Do DIY Strategies Relieve Pain?

We have three sources of information on the effectiveness of DIY strategies. One source is trials in which women were allotted by chance to one form of treatment or another. A review of these trials included trials of hypnosis, immersion in warm water (soaking in a tub or pool deep enough to immerse the belly and big enough to permit moving around), relaxation techniques (progressive muscle relaxation, breathing, Lamaze classes, or yoga), acupressure or acupuncture, and hands-on techniques such as massage or reflexology.[15] The review found that all of these methods did equally well or better at relieving pain, satisfaction with pain relief, or both than their comparison groups (which could be "usual care," a placebo, or a different specific treatment). That tells us that DIY strategies have at least some beneficial effect.

A second source is women themselves. We have two national surveys, one of US women and the other of Canadian women. In the US survey, 67 to 81 percent of respondents rated using a *birth ball* (a large, sturdy exercise ball that can be used for positioning—see Photo 7 above), shower, application of heat or cold, mental strategies such as relaxation, position changes, environmental enhancements such as music, and breathing techniques as "very" or "somewhat" helpful, and 91 percent gave one of these two ratings to immersion in warm water and hands-on techniques such as massage.[10] By comparison, 75 percent rated opioids as "very" or "somewhat" helpful. In the Canadian survey, 72 to 84 percent of respondents rated breathing exercises, position changes, walking, massage, bath or shower, and using a birthing ball as "very" or "somewhat" helpful.[21] By comparison, 59 percent rated N2O inhalation and 62 percent rated opioids as "very" or "somewhat" helpful. In other words, women generally rated DIY strategies as more helpful or at least just as helpful as opioids or N2O inhalation.

Finally, a large study proves that coping with labor using DIY strategies alone is doable: among 8800 women planning birth at home or in *freestanding birth centers* (birth centers independent of a hospital), a mere 3 percent were transferred to hospital care because they wanted an epidural or other pain medication.[18]

WHAT ARE THE ADVANTAGES OF DIY STRATEGIES?

Let's start by looking at the advantages of DIY strategies as a class, move on to what we know about the benefits of specific methods, and wrap up with the research into the use of multiple coping strategies.

WHAT ARE THE BENEFITS OF DIY STRATEGIES AS A CLASS?

- **Their number and variety offer many different options.** DIY strategies are the opposite of "one size fits all." If you try something and don't like it, or it doesn't help, you just move on to something else in your toolbox.

- **They provide immediate relief.** Unlike an epidural, you don't have to wait through the preparation, setup, and administration process, or even for the nurse to get to you with the opioid injection or N2O machine. (The exception might be access to a deep tub or bathing pool if the hospital makes these available.)

- **They can be switched in and out as desired.** If something isn't helping anymore—the fancy word for it is "habituation"—you can try something different. And you may be able to return to the first thing later and have it help again.

- **Several strategies can be used simultaneously.** This enhances effectiveness. (See "What Are the Benefits of Combining Strategies?" below.) You can also add DIY strategies to N2O inhalation or opioids, which may improve their effectiveness.

- **They promote a sense of connection and teamwork with your birth partner and others who may be with you.**[26] Women report feeling cared for and looked after, which they valued.

- **They make possible having an ecstatic, and even an orgasmic, birth.**[9] Not everyone has heard of this possibility, but it makes sense considering that labor and birth involve the same organs and produce the same hormones as making love. (If the topic of orgasmic birth interests you, see #9 in this chapter's reference list for a book on the topic.)

- ***They have no adverse effects!*** This cannot be said of epidurals, opioids, or even N2O inhalation. In fact, as we'll see, the opposite is true. DIY strategies may provide other benefits in addition to moderating pain.

WHAT ARE THE BENEFITS OF SPECIFIC METHODS?

WARM SHOWERS

A trial assigning women to either taking warm showers once they had reached 4 cm dilation or to usual care found that:[16]

- **Warm showers reduce pain.** Women in the showering group gave lower scores to their pain intensity. The difference persisted up to twenty minutes after the shower.

- **Warm showers increase feelings of control.** Women in the showering group gave higher scores on a questionnaire measuring how in charge they felt during the labor.

WARM-WATER IMMERSION

- **Warm-water immersion reduces pain.** A *systematic review* (a study of studies on a particular topic) found that in trials of immersion versus no immersion, women assigned to immersion reported less pain.[7] A national survey of Australian women reporting on their experience with water immersion found that 48 percent of respondents entirely agreed and 25 percent mostly agreed with the statement: "Water immersion was effective pain relief."[8]

Warm-water immersion results in fewer epidurals. The same systematic review as above found that fewer women assigned to immersion had epidurals (39 versus 42 percent).[7] Although small, this difference was "statistically significant," meaning it was unlikely to be due to chance. (If you want to know more about how researchers determine whether differences are probably due to the effects of treatment and not just a chance occurrence, see "Taking a Deeper Dive" at the end of this chapter.)

Moreover, the true difference may be greater than it appears. The trials that produced this data analyzed results according to whether women were *assigned* to immerse, not whether they *actually* immersed, and nearly a quarter of the assigned women didn't. This reduces the pool (sorry, can't resist a pun) of women who experienced immersion's potential benefits. (If you're curious about why results weren't analyzed according to whether women immersed, see "Problems with the Research" in the "Deeper Dive" section of Chapter 2: Epidurals.)

- **Warm-water immersion enhances psychological experience.** The Australian survey reported that more than half of the women engaging in warm-water immersion completely or mostly agreed with the following statements:[8]

"I felt safe." (62 percent entirely agree; 22 percent mostly agree)

"I felt relaxed." (41 percent entirely agree; 26 percent mostly agree)

"Water immersion was soothing." (53 percent entirely agree; 22 percent mostly agree)

"I felt in control." (33 percent entirely agree; 28 percent mostly agree)

"I was able to move freely." (46 percent entirely agree; 26 percent mostly agree)

"I felt protected." (42 percent entirely agree; 22 percent mostly agree)

"I was able to adopt a comfortable position." (37 percent entirely agree; 30 percent mostly agree)

"I felt a sense of privacy." (45 percent entirely agree; 27 percent mostly agree)

In addition, we have a review of *qualitative studies* (studies dealing with words and meanings in order to investigate people's feelings and beliefs about their experiences) in which reviewers looked for common themes in studies interviewing women about their experience of water immersion.[11] Here are some themes that emerged from their analysis, together with illustrating quotes:

Water immersion helped with the pain and enhanced feelings of control:

> *Water softened the whole thing and made it more bearable ... it was much easier to cope with the pain.*

Water immersion increased buoyancy and provided greater freedom of movement:

> *I was really happy to be able to twist and turn and relax [in] the warmth. That is really nice, and you can feel it in your whole body.*

Water immersion enhanced feelings of safety, protection, and privacy:

> *It was like lying in my own womb with the water against my body from all directions, like in a small corner, or nest perhaps.*

Water immersion facilitated a positive state of altered consciousness:

> *Another world ... it was like by the ocean, and then you come back to land, and you are in another country ... They call it 'labourland' ... It really was another world.*

MINDFUL MEDITATION

Mindful meditation is a technique that cultivates paying deliberate and nonjudgmental attention to what is going on physically and emotionally in the moment. Using the technique can increase tolerance and acceptance. A study evaluated whether it could help women experiencing extreme levels of fear of labor and anxiety about labor pain.[27] Investigators assigned women scoring extremely high for these characteristics either to classes training them in mindful meditation or to classes educating them on factors causing fear of labor and helping them plan how to cope. Compared with the classes, mindful meditation training resulted in:

- **fewer women preferring cesarean delivery** (14 versus 53 percent),

- **fewer women having an elective cesarean delivery** (1 versus 12 percent),

- **fewer women having epidurals for labor** (39 versus 59 percent),* and

- **more women having unmedicated births** (42 versus 22 percent).

If mindful meditation could have this major an effect on women with extreme fear of labor, then surely it would be helpful to women experiencing normal levels of anxiety as well.

WHAT ARE THE BENEFITS ACCORDING TO WHETHER THE STRATEGY MODERATES PAIN SENSATION OR PERCEPTION?

We have a review that is complicated to explain, so bear with me because I think it's worth the effort.[5]

Reviewers grouped trials of DIY strategies according to whether the strategy moderated pain sensation or pain perception. Before we dive into the details of the study, let's start with an explanation of what is meant by moderating "pain sensation" versus "pain perception."

Strategies that moderate *pain sensation* work by introducing competing, non-painful sensations to the sensory nerves, which partially blocks transmission of painful sensations. In this category, reviewers put trials of

---

* Rates are lower than you would expect in the US because this study was conducted in the Netherlands, where epidurals are less the norm.

massage, warm-water immersion, position changes and/or walking, using a birth ball for positioning, and warm packs.

Strategies that moderate *pain perception* work by influencing how women think and feel about the pain. They also increase endorphin secretion, the "runner's high" hormone that enables feeling good while also feeling pain. In this category, reviewers put trials of childbirth-preparation classes; continuous support by a woman (e.g., doula, nurse, or female relative); and attention techniques (e.g., hypnosis, music, mental imagery, and aromatherapy).

They took this approach for two reasons. First, trials that evaluate a single strategy often have too few participants even when aggregated to reliably determine whether the strategy has benefits. (See "Taking a Deeper Dive" below to learn why too few participants is an issue.) Pooling data from trials of different strategies that all moderated pain in the same way would increase numbers, potentially solving that problem. Second, grouping trials according to whether they moderated pain sensation or pain perception would avoid inappropriately pooling data from trials that were actually measuring different effects.

Unfortunately for my presenting the review's results, the reviewers didn't provide percentages. What they did provide is odds ratios, which are a way of describing the percent increase or decrease in the probability of a particular outcome in one group compared with its occurrence rate in a different group. (For more about odds ratios, see "Taking a Deeper Dive.") In the case of this review, the odds ratios tell us the effect of pain-modification strategies on outcomes such as cesarean delivery or use of epidurals compared with women receiving "usual care," defined as anything other than the routine use of non-drug pain-relief strategies.[5]

- **Use of strategies moderating pain sensation** resulted in:
  - **Fewer cesarean deliveries.** The odds ratio was 0.61 (39 percent less likely compared with usual care) when data from trials of walking in labor were pooled. However, when data were pooled from all trials of strategies that moderated pain sensation, the odds of cesarean were similar in both groups.

▫ **Less epidural use.** The odds ratio was 0.82 (18 percent less likely compared with usual care) when data were pooled from all trials of strategies that moderated pain sensation.

▫ **Less use of IV oxytocin to augment labor.** The odds ratio was 0.63 (37 percent less likely compared with usual care) when data were pooled from all trials of strategies that moderated pain sensation.

• **Use of strategies moderating pain perception** resulted in:

▫ **Fewer cesarean deliveries.** The odds ratio was 0.57 (43 percent less likely compared with usual care) when data were pooled from all trials of strategies that moderated pain perception. The odds ratio was 0.61 (39 percent less likely compared with usual care) when data were pooled from trials of *continuous labor support* (trials in which women were assigned to have either a member of her social circle, a hospital staff person, or a doula with them continuously or not), and the odds ratio was 0.76 (24 percent less likely compared with usual care) when data were pooled from trials reporting the effect in first-time mothers.

▫ **Fewer instrumental vaginal deliveries.** The odds ratio was 0.83 (17 percent less likely compared with usual care) when data were pooled from all trials of strategies that moderated pain perception. The odds ratio was 0.75 (25 percent less likely compared with usual care) when data were pooled from trials of continuous labor support, and the odds ratio was 0.77 (23 percent less likely compared with usual care) when data were pooled from trials reporting the effect in first-time mothers.

▫ **Less epidural use.** The odds ratio was 0.88 (12 percent less likely compared with usual care) when data were pooled from all trials of strategies that moderated pain perception.

▫ **Less use of IV oxytocin to augment labor.** The odds ratio was 0.83 (17 percent less likely compared with usual care) when data were pooled from all trials of strategies that moderated pain perception, and the odds ratio was 0.76 (24 percent less likely compared with usual care) when data were pooled from trials reporting the effect in first-time mothers.

▫ **Fewer newborns needing resuscitation at birth.** The odds ratio was 0.90 (10 percent less likely compared with usual care) when data were pooled from all trials of strategies that moderated pain perception.

▫ **Greater satisfaction with the childbirth experience.** When data were pooled from all trials of strategies that moderated pain perception, the odds ratio for rating the childbirth experience as positive was 3.45 (almost three and a half times as likely compared with usual care) and for rating it as negative was 0.50 (50 percent less likely compared with usual care).

All in all, the reviewers made 67 comparisons of various outcomes between DIY strategies and usual care in trials overall and in various subgroups, *and not one comparison favored usual care*—although to be fair, some differences favoring DIY strategies may have been due to chance. (See the Deeper Dive section on statistical significance for more information.) It is also worth noting that the benefits of non-drug strategies are probably greater than they appear because "usual care" could also include non-drug strategies for coping with labor pain. Furthermore, typical obstetric management includes routine or frequent use of practices and policies that can increase discomfort or pain, make it difficult to use DIY strategies, or both. These include routine IVs, IV oxytocin to induce or strengthen labor, breaking the bag of waters, forbidding drinking or eating, confinement to bed, and continuous fetal monitoring.

What Are the Benefits of Combining Strategies?

- **Doula care.** Doulas are, in essence, all the DIY components in one package. They supply DIY strategies tailored to the woman's individual needs, plus they provide one-on-one continuous emotional support, a key element of a satisfying birth experience. A systematic review of trials allocating women to care by a doula versus usual care found that doula care resulted in:[2]

- □ **somewhat fewer women having any analgesia** (72 versus 75 percent),

- □ **somewhat fewer women having an epidural** (66 versus 69 percent),

- □ **fewer women having cesareans** (14 versus 21 percent),

- □ **somewhat fewer women having instrumental vaginal deliveries** (18 versus 20 percent), and

- □ **decreased likelihood of dissatisfaction with the birth experience** (12 versus 18 percent).

Some of the differences are small, but statistical analysis shows that they are probably not due to chance.

- ▪ **Learning multiple DIY strategies.** We also have a trial in which investigators assigned women to a childbirth-education class teaching DIY techniques (acupressure, visualization and relaxation, breathing, massage, yoga, and "facilitated partner support") or to usual care.[17] Taking the class resulted in:

- □ **fewer women having an epidural** (24 versus 69 percent),

- □ **fewer women having IV oxytocin to augment labor** (28 versus 58 percent),

- □ **fewer women having cesareans** (18 versus 33 percent), and

- □ **fewer newborns needing resuscitation at birth** (14 versus 29 percent).

Women may also have been less likely to have instrumental vaginal deliveries (14 versus 21 percent), but there were too few participants (171 total) for statistical analysis to reliably determine whether the difference between groups was probably not due to chance. As a sidenote, the investigators theorize that the differences between groups have to do with fewer women having epidurals and thereby avoiding their adverse effects.

- **Combining strategies from the pain-sensation and pain-perception categories.** The review grouping DIY strategies according to whether they modified pain sensation or pain perception also aggregated data from trials that combined at least one strategy from each category.[5] As you can see, using strategies from both categories hits the effectiveness jackpot compared with strategies from either category alone, resulting in:

  ◦ **Fewer cesarean deliveries.** The odds ratio is 0.46 (54 percent less likely) with strategies from both categories versus 0.57 (43 percent less likely) with perception-modification strategies and no reduction with sensation-modification strategies.

  ◦ **Fewer instrumental vaginal deliveries.** The odds ratio is 0.70 (30 percent less likely) with strategies from both categories versus 0.88 (12 percent less likely) with perception-modification strategies and 0.82 (18 percent less likely) with sensation-modification strategies.

  ◦ **Less epidural use.** The odds ratio is 0.46 (54 percent less likely) with strategies from both categories versus 0.57 (43 percent less likely) with perception-modification strategies and no reduction with sensation-modification strategies.

  ◦ **Less use of IV oxytocin to augment labor.** The odds ratio is 0.64 (36 percent less likely) with strategies from both categories versus 0.83 (17 percent less likely) with perception-modification strategies and 0.63 (37 percent less likely) with sensation-modification strategies.

WHAT ARE THE DISADVANTAGES OF DIY STRATEGIES?

As I said in the "Advantages" section, DIY strategies have no adverse effects, but do they have other disadvantages?

- **They don't eradicate pain.** If that's your priority, then you will want to plan for an epidural. Even so, as I said in the introduction,

88

LABOR PAIN: WHAT'S YOUR BEST STRATEGY?

I recommend learning DIY strategies because you will almost certainly find them useful for some part of the labor.

- **They require an investment of time, money, and probably both.** If you are hoping to cope with labor using DIY strategies alone, you will want to set things up in your favor. This may mean finding care providers and a location for birth where philosophy, policies, practices, and resources support your choice because many care providers and hospitals don't. You and your birth partner will need to gain skills and knowledge, which means taking childbirth-education classes aimed at preparing you to cope with labor without meds. Also, you may want to hire a doula who can help support you and your birth partner throughout the birth.

Also, while DIY strategies don't have any harms as a class, are there possible harms connected with specific ones?

- **Warm-water immersion?** One concern is the possibility of uterine or newborn infection, especially if the bag of waters (the bag of amniotic fluid surrounding the baby) has broken. Studies of tub immersion consistently find no increase in infection.[3, 7, 25] In fact, an ingenious study done decades ago proved that bathwater doesn't enter the vagina. Investigators had pregnant women with starch-impregnated tampons immerse in bathwater containing iodine. If water got into the vagina, the iodine would turn the starch purple, but this didn't happen.[23]

  Another concern is maternal fever because high internal temperatures can have an adverse effect on the baby. Immersing in water that is too hot can provoke a fever, but unlike epidural fevers, all you have to do to bring down the fever is get out of the tub.

  Finally, some evidence suggests that warm-water immersion in early labor can slow labor.[7] The solution here is to hold off on immersion until active labor. You may even wish to try a warm bath as a strategy to quiet things down if you are having early contractions that aren't going anywhere but are keeping you from rest or sleep.

- **Skin injury if a heat pack is too hot or ice is applied to bare skin?** This could happen because laboring women tend to be insensitive to heat and cold against their skin, but preventing it is easy. Labor companions need only test the temperature when applying a hot pack and use an intervening cloth when applying ice.

In Summary

The research evidence disconfirms some common assumptions about labor pain, what makes for a positive birth experience, and the effectiveness of DIY strategies. The research finds:

- **Labor pain is a subjective experience.** Whether it is manageable without pain medication depends largely, although not entirely, on intention, expectation, and preparation and the supportive care given by those around the laboring woman.

- **Degree of pain relief and satisfaction with the birth experience don't necessarily correlate.** Degree of pain relief only determines satisfaction when a woman experiences more pain than she personally finds acceptable.

- **DIY strategies are effective at moderating pain.** Combining strategies enhances their effect.

In addition to reducing pain:

- **DIY strategies can increase satisfaction with the birth experience,**

- **DIY strategies can reduce use of medical interventions and improve outcomes, and**

- **DIY strategies have no adverse effects that can't be quickly and easily remedied.**

TAKING A DEEPER DIVE

If all you're looking for is the data you need to make a decision, there's no need to read this section. However, if you've been wondering "What the heck is she talking about?" when I brought up statistical significance, odds ratios, and the importance of study size in the main part of the chapter, settle in. Here's where I'll explain:

- **statistical significance** and why researchers can never rule out that a study result was due to chance,

- **p-values and ratios (odds or risk)**, two methods for ascertaining whether a result is statistically significant, and

- **power,** a calculation that determines how study size impacts statistical significance.

What Does "Statistical Significance" Mean?

Earlier in this chapter, I defined qualitative studies as studies dealing with words and meanings in order to investigate people's feelings and beliefs. Many of the studies we've looked at, though, have been quantitative studies. *Quantitative studies,* as you would surmise, are studies that use numerical measurements to evaluate whether an *intervention* (the variable the researchers are investigating) has an effect on outcomes compared with a *control group* (a group not exposed to the intervention). A crucial question in that evaluation is how likely it is that differing results between the intervention group and the control group were not due to chance. Statistical analysis answers that question.

Notice I said "how likely" not "whether" an effect is due to chance. Statistical analysis can't tell you for certain whether an effect is due to chance. Here's why. Let's suppose you have a theory that flipping a coin with the nondominant hand will increase the number of "heads." You ask 10 right-handed people to flip a coin with their left hand (the intervention group) and another 10 right-handed people to flip a coin with their right hand (the control group). The 10 right-handed coin flips result in 6 "heads" and 4 "tails," pretty close to the half "heads" and half "tails" you would expect by chance. The 10 left-handed coin flips result in 10 heads. Have you proved your theory?

Maybe, maybe not. You could, after all, flip a coin 10 times and get 10 "heads" purely by chance. You could even get 20 heads out of 20 flips, although the odds of that happening by chance would be very small indeed. The odds that the result you saw was due to chance gets smaller and smaller the more it deviates from the expected results, but it never goes to zero.

So, if there is no point at which you can say with complete certainty that the difference between groups wasn't due to chance, where does that leave you? The best you can do is pick a threshold for deciding results are sufficiently unlikely to be due to chance that it's reasonable to conclude something other than chance is influencing the result—hopefully, the intervention, which in this case was flipping the coin with the nondominant hand. You then call results meeting or exceeding that threshold *statistically significant*, meaning results were probably not, but still could have been, due to chance, and you call results failing to meet that threshold *not significant*, meaning they were probably, but not necessarily, due to chance.

The next question becomes: "What is that threshold and how do you calculate whether your results have met it?" That takes us to our next topic.

How Do Researchers Ascertain Statistical Significance?

One way to quantify whether a difference between groups is due to chance is to calculate its *p-value*, p being short for *probability*. By convention, a statistical calculation that finds 5 percent odds (i.e., 1 in 20 odds) or smaller that a difference between groups is due to chance is considered good enough to call the difference statistically significant. Or you could think of it the other way around and say that there is at least a 95-percent probability (i.e., 19 in 20 odds) that the difference *wasn't* due to chance.

Another way to make the calculation is via odds ratios or risk ratios. These involve either dividing the rate of occurrence of an outcome in one group by the rate of occurrence in the other group (*risk ratio*) or dividing the odds of the outcome occurring in one group by the odds of it occurring in the other group (*odds ratio*). Explaining how these work and the differences between them is outside the scope of this book. All you need to know for the purposes of our discussion here is that in both cases, the result of that division tells you the magnitude of the effect of your intervention. For example, as we saw above, a study found that using strategies that moderated pain sensation had an odds ratio of 0.82 for epidural use—meaning that epidural use was 18 percent less likely—compared with usual care.

So once you've calculated the odds ratio or risk ratio, how do you tell if it is statistically significant? That brings us to the confidence interval.

Odds and risk ratios are always accompanied by their *confidence intervals*. The confidence interval is a range around the risk- or odds-ratio value that has a 95-percent probability of containing the true value and a 5-percent probability that it does not. (Note, by the way, that this is the same statistical threshold that applies to p-values.) If all the values within the range are either less than 1 or greater than 1, then the difference between groups was probably not due to chance, that is, it achieves statistical significance. If the range *includes* 1, then one possible value for the ratio is 1/1 = 1, that is, an equal probability of that outcome occurring in both groups, and the result is not statistically significant.

Let's look at a couple of examples to see how this works. A systematic review reported that continuous labor support from a doula (the intervention) versus usual care (the control group) had a risk ratio of 0.61 and a confidence interval of 0.45–0.83 for the outcome of cesarean delivery.[2] That means that compared with usual care, having a doula reduced the probability of cesarean delivery most likely by 39 percent, although the true percent reduction could be as great as 55 percent or as small as 17 percent. We also know the reduction is statistically significant because all the possible values are less than 1. On the other hand, continuous support from a hospital staff member versus usual care had a risk ratio of 0.94 and a confidence interval of 0.84–1.05. That means the reduction was not statistically significant because one of the values in the range of possible values was 1, or no difference between groups. (FYI: When I gave you the odds ratios for pain-sensation and pain-perception strategies above, I left out the confidence intervals. However, I only gave you odds ratios for comparisons that were statistically significant.)

So far, we've talked about what statistical significance means and two ways to establish it: p-values and odds or risk ratios. Now let's talk about the importance of "power."

WHAT IS A POWER CALCULATION?

The ability to determine statistical significance depends on the number of events being measured—how many times the coin was flipped, if you like. The larger the number, the more reliable the determination that the deviance from what was expected probably wasn't due to chance. This is because the greater the number of events, the more the results tend toward the average.

Let's go back to our original coin-flipping example. You remember that in our control group, 10 right-handed people flipped a coin with their right hand. In our intervention group, another 10 right-handed people flipped a coin with their left hand. The 10 right-handed coin flips resulted in 6 "heads" and 4 "tails," which wasn't far off what you would expect by chance, and the 10 left-handed flips resulted in 10 "heads" and 0 "tails," which would seem unusual but not off the charts. But what if we had 100 right-handed people flipping right-handed and getting 60 heads and 40 tails and 100 right-handed people flipping left-handed and getting 100 heads? The 60/40 split would seem nothing out of the way, but 100 heads out of 100 flips? Those are the same percentages as in the first example, but surely, you would be thinking that something was almost certainly influencing the fall of the coins (although, of course, you could still be looking at a chance event).

Power calculations answer the question: "How many participants do we need in this study in order to have reasonable odds of detecting a significant difference between the group having the intervention and the control group? To answer it, investigators start with how often an outcome they consider important occurs in the control group (the *primary outcome*). Next, they estimate the effect they think the intervention they're studying will have on that outcome. Then they use those numbers to calculate the number of people needed in the study in order to have a reasonable probability of detecting a significant difference. For reasons having to do with the practicalities of conducting research, investigators usually shoot for a number of participants that will give an 80-percent probability of detecting whether the difference in the primary outcome is statistically significant.

If the study has too few participants to have a good chance of finding a significant difference, the study is considered *underpowered*. Studies can be underpowered for any number of reasons. The investigators may not have been able to recruit as many participants as they planned, or participants may have been lost to follow-up. The study may be powered to detect a difference in the primary outcome but not other outcomes that are also of interest but occur less frequently. For example, a study might be powered to detect a difference in the percentage of newborns born in poor condition as measured by low Apgar scores or low umbilical-cord blood pH but be *underpowered* to detect differences in newborn mortality, which would occur much more rarely.

Failing to find a significant difference in underpowered studies doesn't rule out the possibility of an effect. It just means the jury is still out.

TWO FINAL POINTS ABOUT STATISTICAL SIGNIFICANCE

Because you are dealing with probabilities, not certainties, there is always the possibility that an outcome that fails to achieve statistical significance isn't due to chance. The reverse is also true: it is always possible, however unlikely, that an outcome that achieves statistical significance is due to chance.

With one possible exception, the only studies that can show causation are trials that randomly allocate participants to the intervention or control group. This is because allocating people by chance eliminates the possibility that differences in outcomes are attributable to differences in the participants rather than the intervention. All other study types can only show associations. This is because, despite applying statistical techniques to account for factors that differ between groups and could explain differences in outcomes, there is always the possibility of unknown factors or factors that weren't considered. The possible exception to this rule may be propensity score analyses. (See "Taking a Deeper Dive" in Chapter 2.)

Chapter 7:
Your Take-Away

Hopefully, if you're reading this chapter, it's because you've gotten what you need to determine how you plan to cope with the pain of labor. Good for you! Now let's see what I can do to help you implement your plan in a way that maximizes the pros of your chosen strategy while minimizing its cons.

As I see it, the road forks according to your decision either to make epidural analgesia "Plan A" or to make it "Plan B." It makes sense, then, to divide the chapter into two main sections based on this choice.

So, here's the setup:

"An Epidural Is 'Plan A'" takes what we've learned about epidural drawbacks and offers ways to avoid or mitigate them so that you have an optimal epidural experience.

"An Epidural Is 'Plan B'" covers how to plan for an experience that supports having an unmedicated birth. In the typical hospital, this may not be as easy as you might think, and we'll talk about why not in this section too. The "Plan B" section will also cover navigating a switch to an epidural in midlabor in a way that promotes feeling satisfied with your decision in the long term.

In addition, as we've seen, you have two additional options that fall between epidurals and DIY strategies: opioids and nitrous oxide (N2O) inhalation. To address these, I'll include a subsection in both main sections on how opioids and N2O inhalation might fit in with your overall plan.

Also, regardless of which path you plan to take, it would be wise to learn about some of the aspects of the other choice.

If an epidural is "Plan A," I recommend that you take childbirth-preparation classes that teach DIY strategies. Here's why:

- You may need DIY strategies while you are still at home.

- If you wish to delay an epidural until active labor, a strategy that can reduce the likelihood of some of its problems, you will need ways to cope during that time.

- The anesthesiologist may not be available when you are ready for your epidural.

- You will need coping strategies to get through the time it can take to prepare you for the epidural, administer it, and have it take effect.

- You may be among the roughly 10 percent of women who don't find an epidural helpful or helpful enough.[11, 19, 34]

- It is possible that labor will turn out to be easier than you thought, and you may decide you don't want an epidural after all.

On the other hand, if you're making an epidural "Plan B," I recommend that you review the strategies for optimizing an epidural covered under "An

Epidural Is 'Plan A'." As I wrote earlier, things don't always go according to plan. You don't want to cross an epidural off your dance card.

A final thought before we dive in: both "An Epidural Is 'Plan A'" and "An Epidural Is 'Plan B'" start with choosing care providers and a location for birth. However, you may be far enough along in pregnancy that you've already made these choices. I strongly recommend that you check out whether you've got the right people and location anyway. If you have, great! You can breathe a sigh of relief. If the situation isn't optimal, but it's acceptable, that's good to know too. You won't be disappointed or unpleasantly surprised, and you can start thinking about how you might work the system in your favor. If you really haven't got the right people or place, and it's at all possible to switch, I urge you to make the effort. A lot is riding on this. Don't stay where you are and hope for the best. You might get lucky, but the odds are against it. Finally, if you have no better option or can't make a switch, it's better to know now and start thinking about how you might cope with the problems that might arise than to go in eyes shut thinking there won't be any.

Tip: I suggest you bookmark this chapter (if you are reading this as an e-book) or copy it and bring it with you to the birth (if you have purchased a hard copy). Having it to refer to may come in handy in labor.

AN EPIDURAL IS "PLAN A"

As I wrote in the introduction, if you're planning an epidural, your task is to set yourself up for an optimal epidural experience. Here are my suggestions for how to do that along with the reasons for each suggestion.

- **Choose a midwife or doctor with a low cesarean surgery rate.** This is the most important choice you can make, especially if this is your first baby. As I wrote in the epidural chapter, your probability of having a cesarean depends more on your care provider's philosophy and practices than on whether you have an epidural, or, for that matter, on pretty much anything that has to do with you. A nonconfrontational way of asking a doctor or midwife their cesarean rate is: "How often do you find it necessary to do a cesarean?"

As for what's a good cesarean rate in a mixed population of women having first babies, women with previous vaginal births, and women with previous cesareans, research has found that the sweet spot is between 10 and 15 percent.[16] You aren't likely to find an obstetrician these days with rates that low—the US cesarean rate is 32 percent and has been for over a decade—but I'd take anything above the low 20 percents as a red flag. A midwife's rate should be substantially lower as they only take clients at low risk for cesarean.

The catch is that almost all doctors and midwives work in group practices and rotate call for attending births, and members of the same practice may have widely differing rates. And in some cases, staff obstetricians called *hospitalists* may manage all deliveries, which means the people you see in pregnancy won't be attending the birth. If it's a small practice, you can ask everyone, and if it's a hospitalist situation, you can ask the hospital the average rate.

- **Here's what to look for in a hospital:**

  - **The hospital can handle obstetric emergencies 24/7.** Not every hospital has this capacity, and as we have seen, epidurals can sometimes cause problems that require an urgent response and the ability to deal with serious complications. To handle emergencies, the hospital should have 24/7 obstetric, pediatric, and anesthesia staff on duty and at least a *Level II nursery*, that is, a nursery capable of caring for newborns with moderate problems and stabilizing sicker babies for transport to a hospital with a neonatal intensive-care unit.

  - **Epidurals are readily available 24/7.** Some hospitals may not have in-house anesthesia staff at night.

  - **Anesthesiologists allow your support people to be present during the epidural administration procedure.**[29] Not all anesthesiologists permit the presence of a birth partner or doula, and you will want them with you. The administration procedure will be a stressful time as you will have to hold absolutely still, and you will undoubtedly have one or more contractions before the anesthesiologist is finished.

   ▫ **The hospital has breastfeeding-friendly policies (if you're planning on breastfeeding).**[13, 20, 35] As we saw, epidurals may cause problems with breastfeeding. A hospital with breastfeeding-friendly policies can help compensate for that. Breastfeeding-friendly policies include healthy mothers and babies kept together after birth, breastfeeding initiation within the first hour, twenty-four-hour rooming-in, no bottles, no pacifiers, nursing staff trained in how to assist breastfeeding moms, and access to a breastfeeding specialist.

- **If the cost of the birth is an issue for you, find out how much an epidural costs so you can plan accordingly.** Out-of-pocket epidural costs may run as high as three thousand dollars and may be substantial even if you have insurance.[4, 9]

- **Consider hiring a doula.** You may wish to have a doula for the same reasons I suggested earlier that you learn DIY strategies. In addition:

   ▫ A doula will have ideas and strategies for helping labor progress in women with epidurals.

   ▫ Even if you are free of pain, you may still benefit from emotional support and encouragement. It's unlikely that nursing staff will play this role. Even when women aren't medicated, nurses usually spend very little time in the room,[14, 15, 27] and when in the room, they don't spend much time providing supportive care.[28] Moreover, most nurses see their job as managing your pain.[6, 15, 23] This means that once you have an epidural, most nurses will see your need for supportive care as having been met.

   ▫ You will have someone in your corner to help you work through decisions that you may need to make and to help you get the information you need to make them.

- **Consider delaying an epidural until at least 5 cm dilation.** One reason to delay an epidural until active labor is that starting an epidural in early labor may increase the odds of having a cesarean. The research is muddy on this point, though. Some studies have found that having an epidural in early labor increases the cesarean rate,[22, 25, 44] while others didn't find a difference.[42] Additionally, some of the studies finding no difference are flawed. In several of them, epidurals were mostly administered around the same point in dilation. Other studies that showed no difference, though, seem sound.[17] Many obstetricians will tell you that epidural timing doesn't matter; I don't think an effect has been ruled out.

All that said, delaying an epidural still has two benefits. First, because the probability of epidural-related fever rises with epidural duration, delaying an epidural helps avoid developing a fever and therefore the consequences of fever.[26] Second, the adverse effects of the opioid in the anesthetic mixture may be dose-related. That means that delaying an epidural will reduce the amount of anesthetic you receive over the course of the labor, which in turn may help avoid problems with breastfeeding.[5] (See the epidural chapter for a more detailed discussion.)

- **Go straight to an epidural.** Don't try an opioid first. The effects of the IV or injected opioid and the epidural opioid are additive.[1] Remifentanil may be the exception to this because it is metabolized so rapidly.[46] You may wish to ask which opioid you would be given should you want it.

- **Choose a standard epidural over a combined spinal-epidural.** As we saw in the combined spinal-epidural chapter, CSEs offer no advantages, and they increase the likelihood of unpleasant side effects. *Warning*: If you do opt for a CSE, become very sleepy, and cannot be roused, your birth partner should get help immediately. As we discussed in the chapter on CSEs, they can depress respiration, sometimes severely.

- **Stay off your back, even semi-reclining.** On your back, gravity tends to hold an *occiput posterior* (facing your belly) baby in that unfavorable position. Seated upright and leaning forward, side-lying, and turned three-quarters over (*semi-prone*) positions encourage babies to take up and maintain the favorable position facing your back.[39]

- **Make sure that you don't get into awkward positions and that you change positions every half hour if you are awake.**[38] Being numb will prevent you from feeling the discomfort that normally tells you to shift position and could lead later to aches, pains, or even injury. Likewise, you won't feel pain from pressure so make sure to pad the bed rail with a pillow if you are lying against it or put a pillow between your legs if you are side-lying.

- **If body temperature begins rising, cool down.** Your support people can remove blankets, wipe you down with cool cloths, fan you, etc.[38] It may help, and it can't hurt.

- **Push like a woman without an epidural who is pushing instinctively.** You may be coached to hold your breath and bear down as long and hard as you can, but waiting for the contraction to build, bearing down for five to seven seconds, taking four to six quick breaths, and repeating throughout the contraction will likely be equally effective and should put less stress on your pelvic floor.[38]

- **Push side-lying or in an upright position.** Pushing in positions other than reclining or semi-reclining is generally more effective and having an epidural need not prevent you from assuming them. You may need assistance with your top leg for side-lying and "spotters" for positions such as a squat or kneeling upright, but with today's modern, light epidurals, most women have enough muscle strength and control to assume these positions with assistance or even without it.

- **If someone is helping you with your legs during pushing, make sure they don't hold them in exaggerated or awkward positions.** Again, with an epidural, you won't feel the discomfort that ordinarily would signal impending back, joint, or nerve injury.

- **Decline a cesarean or instrumental delivery based solely on exceeding a time limit.**[8] It isn't uncommon to base the decision to deliver the baby on a "one size fits all" time limit rather than considering the individual situation, e.g.: Is progress being made? How are mother and baby doing? What has been tried to facilitate progress? Epidurals can lengthen labor. Having more time improves your chances of birthing on your own.

- **If you experience a post-dural-puncture headache, an epidural blood patch can be helpful in both the short and long terms.** A *post-dural-puncture headache* is a severe headache that occurs when the epidural needle accidentally pierces the dural membrane. This allows the cerebrospinal fluid to leak out, and the ensuing drop in cerebrospinal fluid pressure causes the headache. An *epidural blood patch* is a procedure in which a small amount of your blood is injected into the epidural space close to the puncture site to clot and seal the leak. It almost always relieves the headache (90 percent),[21] and it has also been found to reduce the percentage of women subsequently experiencing recurrent headaches, severe headaches, and probably chronic backache as well.[30, 45]

Dural puncture is not currently recognized as a possible cause of recurrent headache or chronic backache. (See the "Deeper Dive" in the epidural chapter for the research on this point.) If you decide to seek medical help for new or worsened headaches or backaches after having an epidural, it is likely that your doctor won't know that dural puncture is a possible cause. You may wish to discuss this possibility with your doctor as it could affect your diagnosis and management.

- **Have patience if breastfeeding doesn't get off to a good start. Get professional help if you need it.**

HOW MIGHT OPIOIDS AND N2O FIT IN WITH YOUR PLAN?

N2O inhalation might help you hold off on an epidural until active labor. N2O might also be helpful if you are needing something to tide you over until the epidural can be administered. N2O's ability to reduce anxiety might be especially helpful in this latter situation. The problem with N2O inhalation, though, is access. In the US, at least, not that many hospitals offer it. Find out if yours does ahead of time, and if it does, you may want to ask for it when you check into your room to be sure you have it available if you decide you want it.

Opioids can help in these same circumstances, but they have a significant drawback: as we have discussed, the likelihood of your baby experiencing an opioid-related adverse effect increases with the amount of opioid in your system, and epidurals contain opioids too. Remifentanil is a possible exception to this caveat because it is rapidly metabolized.

AN EPIDURAL IS "PLAN B"

This brings us to the other path: you've decided to make an epidural "Plan B." If this is your choice, you have two tasks: one is to structure your experience to maximize your chances of avoiding an epidural, and the other is to develop a strategy for changing your mind during labor. However, before we get to my suggestions for you on these points, I want to talk more about the context in which you will be working because, as I wrote in the introduction, achieving an unmedicated birth in the typical hospital may not be easy or straightforward. Let's start, then, with a look at why this might be so.

WHY COULD AVOIDING AN EPIDURAL BE DIFFICULT?

You would think that hospital staff would be neutral on whether you choose to have or avoid an epidural, but this is often not the case. In the typical hospital, financial considerations and approach to pain management promote preference for you to have an epidural.

Let's look in more detail at those factors and how they can shape provision of care:

- **Economic incentives promote epidural use.** Maintaining a 24/7 dedicated obstetric anesthesia service is desirable, but it's expensive, and it's financed by reimbursement for each procedure. That means the hospital wants to spread out the cost over as many procedures as possible. In addition, having women in bed and not in need of supportive care reduces staffing by permitting monitoring of vital signs and fetal status from a central station.

   While there may be problems with high epidural usage, in the presence of our nursing shortages and economic or business considerations, having a woman in bed, attached to an intravenous line and continuous electronic fetal monitor and in receipt of an epidural may be the only realistic way to go.

   — Anesthesiologist[24]

- **The care goal is to relieve pain, and epidurals do the best job at that.**[6, 7, 15, 40]

   As a nurse, you feel … I want to give you something, so you don't feel bad. So [RNs] carry this with labor. You're in pain? I want to give you the epidural.

   — Nurse [23]

- **With epidurals being the norm,**[37] **care management is often organized on the presumption that women will be in bed and not in need of supportive care.**[6]

   Once they have [had] an epidural … they're actually easier to take care of because they're not hurting. You don't have to be right by their side all the time and they can just fall asleep.

   — Nurse[6]

- **With epidurals being the norm, few nurses are trained to work with unmedicated women, which can increase their reluctance to do so.**[6]

    A barrier to providing supportive care is education of the nurse. Many of the nurses could be better trained in therapies: What to do to help with their [patient's] comfort level and what to do when they hit certain stages.

    — Nurse[6]

- **The needs and care of women who don't have an epidural make extra demands on nursing staff and disrupt usual care routines, which can breed resentment.**

    It's almost like ... they think, "Just get an epidural because I'm not here to babysit you."

    — Nurse[6]

- **Obstetricians tend to prefer the greater predictability and control epidurals provide.**

    By far the most pleasant events for all involved are those where the patients agree to an appropriately timed epidural, and then allow us to alert the patient when it's time to push.

    — Obstetrician[18]

Staff preference for women to have epidurals can create resistance to your not having one. A national US survey reported that nearly one in five respondents reported pressure in labor to agree to an epidural.[12]

    I felt like I was scolded like a child to take the epidural. I cried but eventually gave in.

    — Respondent to a survey[12]

Beyond staff preference, you have another challenge:

- **Typical obstetric management prevents the use of alternative pain-coping strategies.**

    If we put women in hospitals with restrictive policies—they're hooked up to everything, they're expected to be in bed—of course they're going to go for the epidural because they're unable to work through their pain …

    — Nursing professor[3]

All of this is to say that you have your work cut out for you if your plan is to avoid an epidural. It is not to say, though, that it can't be done. Let's look at how you might overcome the obstacles.

How Do You Game the System in Your Favor?

As we have seen, in the typical hospital, you may find yourself swimming upstream against hospital staff pressure, subtle or not so subtle, to have an epidural and in an environment where practices and policies aren't conducive to unmedicated birth. Here are some ideas on how to avoid that problem:

- **Choose a hospital that provides amenities that support a drug-free labor and the policies that go with them.** Amenities would be deep tubs or showers; options for positioning other than lying in bed such as birth balls or rocking chairs; rice socks that can be heated in a microwave; ice packs; and access to pleasant places to walk. Policies would be freedom to eat and drink; IVs only for delivering meds or for women who can't keep liquids down; intermittent listening to the fetal heart rate instead of continuous fetal monitoring; and nurses trained in non-drug strategies.

- **If you are at low risk for complications in labor, consider having your baby in a freestanding birth center—if one is available in your community—or at home.** One way of solving the problem of swimming upstream is to get out of the stream. In the US, be sure to choose a midwife who is certified by either the American College of Nurse-Midwives or the North American Registry of Midwives. The former will have CNM or LM after their name and the latter will have CPM.

- **Choose care providers whose default approach is to support the natural process.** As a bonus, this also ensures that their attitude toward epidurals will align with yours. (FYI: Midwives are more likely to—but don't necessarily—take this approach.)

Medical management—frequent use of induction and augmentation of labor, routine use of IVs, continuous fetal monitoring, confinement to bed, forbidding oral intake—increases pain and discomfort, making it harder to avoid an epidural, while at the same time limiting options for coping with pain. For example, we know that most labor inductions are avoidable because they are done for reasons other than medical indications and that many medical-management practitioners augment labors far more often than they need to.[2] We also know that being induced or augmented is strongly associated with abandoning N2O in favor of an epidural.[31]

- **Ask for the nurse who is most comfortable working with a woman who wants to avoid pain medication.** Repeat your request at each shift change. You may wish to ask your birth partner or doula to remind you to do this as you may be deep into labor and not notice. (If you're wondering why your birth partner or doula can't take care of this for you, messages about your preference to avoid pain medication should come from you. Otherwise, nurses may think your birth partner or doula is expressing their own wishes, not yours.)

- **Tell the nurse please don't ask you if you want pain medication; if you want it, you will let her know.** It's not like you don't know it's available, and the reminder (1) can get you thinking about meds and (2) covertly conveys that it is something you need. One thing you might do is add that you would be grateful to have any advice or help she can give with ideas to increase your comfort and relieve pain that don't involve drugs. As I've been saying, most labor nurses see relieving pain as a primary responsibility. Adding the second part lets nurses know how they still can be of help.

HOW DO YOU PREPARE FOR AN UNMEDICATED LABOR?

The previous section should help avoid problems with the system. On the personal side, you need to be well prepared to cope with labor. Also, you want your birth partner and any others who will be with you to be on the same page as you. Here are some actions you can take to prepare and to ensure that you and your birth partner (and any other labor-support companions) work as a team:

- **Make sure you and your birth partner and any other family or friends who will be with you are willing to back your decision regardless of their opinion about what you should do.** You will be vulnerable in labor, and you don't want pressure in either direction.

- **Hire a doula.** Even if your nurses are neutral to your plan to avoid an epidural, it is doubtful they will provide supportive care. Nurses usually spend very little time in the room with you,[14, 15, 27] and even when they are with you, they don't spend much of that time providing supportive care.[28] Nurses' primary responsibilities are monitoring you and your baby, assisting doctors in performing procedures, and enforcing hospital policies.[15, 32, 41] Supportive care generally comes last if it comes in at all.[10, 33, 41] Doulas fill that gap. They offer ideas to help make you more comfortable and promote labor progress, assist your birth partner and other labor companions with the physical tasks of supporting you through labor, and provide emotional support both to you and to them. However, as with your birth partner and your friends and family, make sure the doula you're considering is prepared to back you in whatever you decide in labor.

- **Take a childbirth-preparation class series that trains you to cope with labor using DIY strategies and prepares you to be a full participant in all decisions.** I suggest this even if you're hiring a doula. A doula acts as a guide, assistant, and on-the-spot expert resource; however, you and your birth partner will still need knowledge and coping skills to work most effectively with your doula.

As to what you're looking for in childbirth-preparation classes:

◻ **Seek out a certified teacher.** This doesn't guarantee excellence, but it's at least a benchmark of having met competency criteria.

◻ **Look for an independent class.** It's a fact of life that childbirth educators have to please the people who pay them and that should be you, not a hospital or clinic. Hospital- or clinic-based classes can be problematic for this reason. They may not teach you DIY strategies because the assumption is that you will be having an epidural.[43] They may also focus on explaining the practices and policies of their institution rather than educating you on the pros and cons of your options.

◻ **Find a series with something on the order of ten to twelve hours of instruction spread out over several weeks.** You can't learn all that you and your birth partner need to know, much less master it, in a few hours or a weekend workshop.

◻ **Look for classes with four to ten couples.** You want a class that's big enough for good discussions and the chance to hear differing points of view or questions you may not have thought of, but small enough to ensure the instructor's individual attention.

HOW DO YOU STRUCTURE A DECISION-MAKING PROCESS FOR CHANGING YOUR MIND IN LABOR?

Whatever you ultimately choose during labor, I want you to come out of the experience feeling good about yourself and your decision-making process. Here are some ways to help you do that:

- **Make your plan to avoid an epidural an intention rather than a goal.** An *intention* focuses on the path. It allows you to prepare while understanding that circumstances may send you in a different direction. A *goal*, by contrast, focuses on the result and whether you succeed or fail in achieving it. An intention allows you to change your mind without judgment.

- **Consider ahead of time how you will handle disappointing news.** Finding out that they hadn't progressed as far as they thought they had led some women to decide to have an epidural.[47] What would you want from your support people if this were to happen to you? There isn't a right choice here. You just want to make a decision that will satisfy you in the long run and avoid an in-the-moment choice that could leave you wondering about it later.

- **Don't make a decision about pain medication in the middle of a contraction.** You are more likely to regret a decision made impulsively in response to contraction pain.

- **Preset some reasonable amount of time, say half an hour or five contractions, that starts if you say you want an epidural.** Your labor companions then have that amount of time to try to help you get more comfortable. At the end of the time, either something they suggested will have worked, you will have gotten past the rough patch, or you still want an epidural, in which case you get it.

- **Alternatively, decide on a code word or phrase.** Provided you don't use it, you can complain, moan, curse, yell, cry—do anything you need to do to vent your feelings—but the moment you use it, you get your epidural, no questions asked.

- **Let your care team know that you would like your dilation to be checked right before going ahead with an epidural.** It can take as much as an hour to administer the IV fluid and prep for the epidural—not to mention that the anesthesiologist might not be available when you make your request. You may have progressed in that time and knowing whether you have or haven't may change your decision.

- **Beware of staff remarks with a hidden barb.** Let's suppose you've decided that you've given it your all but that it's time for an epidural. Shortly after you make your request, the anesthesiologist bops in, grins, and says something like: "Now we'll see some smiles!" or "I think natural childbirth makes about as much sense as natural dentistry." From their point of view, you've come to your senses and affirmed their opinion that an epidural is the only rational way to go, but your perspective and experience may be quite different. Forewarned is forearmed. Alert your birth partner and labor companions to this possibility so that they don't fall in line with it. Your team can best help by affirming your decision-making process. They can, for example, remind you of everything you tried and how hard you worked and, if you're feeling sad or disappointed by the need to change plans, validate those feelings by commiserating with you about it.

HOW MIGHT OPIOIDS AND N2O FIT IN WITH YOUR PLAN?

N2O inhalation could make a good addition to your toolkit if you're planning on avoiding an epidural, especially in light of its psychological effects of easing anxiety and helping you relax. If this option appeals to you, make sure your hospital has it available because while it is growing in popularity, it still isn't common in US hospitals. If it is available, you might want to ask for it as soon as you are admitted even if you don't want to use it right away. Chances are that the hospital doesn't have machines for every labor room, and you don't want to be shut out later because they're all in use. Getting one before you're wanting to use it will also allow you to learn how to manage it and to make sure the machine is working properly.[36]

I can think of one situation where you might want to give opioids a shot (pun intended): you can manage contractions, but you're experiencing unremitting, severe back pain. From my work as a doula back before epidurals became quite so universal, I can tell you that opioids seemed to help with back pain, and that was sometimes enough to keep going without an epidural. You're in luck if the hospital's opioid of choice is remifentanil. Because it is metabolized so rapidly, it is least likely to have adverse effects on the baby.[46] Otherwise, my advice is that if you've decided you want something for pain, go straight to an epidural. As we saw in the opioid chapter, opioids don't do any better at relieving pain than what you've already been doing, plus they have potential adverse effects. Epidurals have them too, but you get your money's worth in pain relief in exchange.

IN SUMMARY

The initial fork in the road is whether you are making an epidural "Plan A" or "Plan B." Regardless of which path you choose:

- You will benefit by knowing the strategies of the other path.

- Your choice of care provider and location for birth are the most important decisions you can make for determining whether you have an optimal experience.

- N2O inhalation may fit in with your plan; opioids may too, but they have disadvantages compared with N2O.

If you are making an epidural "Plan A":

- You have numerous strategies that can help you avoid experiencing an epidural's disadvantages.

If you are making an epidural "Plan B":

- You may need to take action to minimize opposition from hospital staff and to obtain care that is conducive to unmedicated birth.

- Take a childbirth-preparation class series that trains you to cope with labor using DIY strategies and teaches you the pros and cons of your options.

- Your birth partner and any other family members or friends who will be present must be prepared to support you in your endeavor.

- Having a process for changing your mind in labor can help you make a decision you will be satisfied with in the long term.

Chapter 8:
My Final Thoughts

I've saved this for last because I wanted to present you the facts as I know them as neutrally as I could so that you could make up your own mind. At this point, though, you've got the information you need to make your own decision. It no longer feels inappropriate to express my opinion, and I'd like to take the opportunity to do that in case you find it useful. Here, then, is what I think:

I think that while an epidural can be a blessing for some labors, there are both pragmatic and experiential reasons for making an epidural "Plan B."

My pragmatic reasons are these:

- **If you can manage without an epidural, why run the risk of possibly experiencing its harms?** Some non-drug options even offer a "twofer": they promote good progress in addition to reducing pain.

- **An epidural may relieve pain yet still leave you suffering.** You may be itchy or nauseous. You may be feeling neglected by staff or loved ones. You or your baby may be experiencing alarming symptoms. You are at greater risk of an instrumental and possibly a surgical delivery, both of which can cause emotional trauma.

- **You can always change your mind and have an epidural,** *but you can't go back.* Well, you could let it wear off, but it would mean taking back the labor pain probably at a more advanced stage having lost your own natural pain-relieving endorphins.

My other reason is more personal:

To repeat what I wrote in the "Deeper Dive" section of the epidural chapter, the dominant model for birth in our culture is that it is a medical process to be managed by drugs and procedures and accomplished as efficiently and painlessly as possible. But there is another model: I know from the stories of others, my work as a doula, and my personal experience that birth can be a rite of passage. Speaking to my personal experience, I found that in meeting labor's challenges, guided by people whose knowledge and wisdom I trusted and supported by my loved ones, labor became a transformational emotional, psychological, and spiritual event that profoundly changed how I thought of myself, my capacities, and my body forever. Because of this possibility, another reason to make an epidural "Plan B" is:

- **You increase the odds of satisfaction with the birth and open the door to the potential for a peak experience.**

That being said, my primary goal in writing this book remains giving you the ability to decide what is right for you and giving you your best shot at obtaining it. Whatever your choice, let it be what you think is best and not what anyone else thinks you should do—including me.

Tables:
Comparing Pain-Relief Methods

DEGREE OF PAIN RELIEF	
Epidurals	Can completely relieve pain
CSE	Can completely relieve pain
Opioids	Modest to moderate pain relief
N2O	Modest to moderate pain relief
DIY	Modest to moderate pain relief

LAG TIME TO PAIN RELIEF	
Epidurals	Time lag from request to relief can take an hour or more
CSE	Same as an epidural
Opioids	Time lag between request and relief is short, provided a nurse responds promptly to the request
N2O	Once the device is set up, relief is immediate
DIY	Relief is immediate; exception: water immersion requires filling a tub

EFFECT ON CONSCIOUSNESS & PSYCHOLOGICAL STATE	
Epidurals	No effect on consciousness; enables the ability to relax, engage with people, and enjoy the birth
CSE	Same as an epidural
Opioids	Sedating
N2O	Can reduce anxiety, help with relaxation, and distract from pain
DIY	No effect on consciousness; promotes a sense of being cared for and looked after; warm-water immersion can enhance the psychological experience

SIDE EFFECTS	
Epidurals	Nausea: 10% Itching: 3% Maternal low blood pressure: 30–40% Fever: 22% Urinary retention: 18% Post-dural-puncture headache: 1% Long-term recurrent headache or backache: < 1%
CSE	Compared with an epidural: Nausea: Same as an epidural Itching: 50% vs. 30% (Note: Trials of epidurals vs. CSEs report much higher itching rates than trials of planned epidural vs. avoided epidural) Maternal low blood pressure requiring treatment: 6% vs. 3% Post-dural-puncture headache: 1% No data on other side effects but presumably the same as an epidural
Opioids	Nausea: 20% Itching: 3–6%
N2O	Nausea: 6% Dizziness: 8% However, clears rapidly from the system when use is discontinued
DIY	None

SEVERE/LIFE-THREATENING EFFECTS	
Epidurals	High blockade or systemic toxic reaction: 2–7 per 10,000 Nerve injury: 1 in 2,600 to 1 in 220,000
CSE	No data on CSEs but presumably the same as an epidural
Opioids	None
N2O	None
DIY	None

EFFECT ON MODE OF DELIVERY	
Epidurals	Instrumental vaginal delivery: A minimum of 4 more first-time mothers per 100; the excess may fall in the range of 9–19 more first-time mothers per 100 Cesarean surgery: An effect is disputed; however, well-conducted studies in women at low risk for cesarean report excess cesarean rates of 6–12 per 100
CSE	Compared with an epidural: Instrumental vaginal delivery: Similar to epidural Cesarean surgery: At best, similar rates and a possible increase; two small trials investigating the effect of episodes of slowed fetal heart rate (see "Adverse Effects on Baby") reported cesarean rates of 9% vs. 2% for this reason
Opioids	No effect on mode of delivery
N2O	No effect on mode of delivery
DIY	Walking can reduce cesarean deliveries; having a doula can reduce cesareans and instrumental vaginal deliveries

EFFECT ON THE BABY	
Epidurals	5-minute Apgar score < 7: 9 more babies per 1000 whose mothers had an epidural (20 vs. 11 per 1000) Admission to intensive-care nursery: 3 more babies per 1000 (7 vs. 4 per 1000) Neurologic symptoms or seizure: 2 per 1000 babies whose mothers ran fevers in labor Breastfeeding: Evidence supports an adverse effect on establishing breastfeeding
CSE	Compared with an epidural: Slowing of the baby's heart rate during labor (bradycardia): 10% vs. 4% No data on other effects on the baby but presumably the same as an epidural
Opioids	Requiring naloxone (Narcan) at birth: 2–15%, depending on the opioid and method of administration; remifentanil may be the exception Requiring resuscitation: 4–14%, depending on the opioid and method of administration; no data for remifentanil
N2O	None
DIY	None

MISCELLANEOUS PROBLEMS	
Epidurals	Epidurals require a package of practices intended to prevent, monitor for, and counteract the epidural's potential adverse effects, all of which have potential adverse effects Epidurals interfere with the production of hormones that regulate breastfeeding, mediate the woman's experience of labor, and influence her maternal feelings toward the baby
CSE	Adverse effects arising from injecting opioids in Stage 1 of the CSE: Difficulty swallowing: 2% Slowed maternal respiration: 6%
Opioids	Opioids interfere with the production of hormones that regulate breastfeeding, mediate the woman's experience of labor, and influence her maternal feelings toward the baby
N2O	N/A
DIY	DIY strategies are difficult to use effectively with usual management in the typical hospital environment

COST	
Epidurals	Costs may run as high as $3,000 even with insurance
CSE	Same as an epidural
Opioids	Unknown but probably modest
N2O	Unknown but probably modest
DIY	May be nil to several thousand dollars if strategies include hiring a doula and taking childbirth-preparation classes

References

CHAPTER 2: EPIDURALS

1. Al Wattar BH, Honess E, Bunnewell S, et al. Effectiveness of intrapartum fetal surveillance to improve maternal and neonatal outcomes: a systematic review and network meta-analysis. CMAJ 2021;193(14):E468-E77.

2. Alehagen S, Wijma B, Lundberg U, et al. Fear, pain and stress hormones during childbirth. J Psychosom Obstet Gynaecol 2005;26(3):153-65.

3. Anim-Somuah M, Smyth RM, Cyna AM, et al. Epidural versus non-epidural or no analgesia for pain management in labour. Cochrane Database Syst Rev 2018;5:CD000331.

4. Ansari JR, Barad M, Shafer S, et al. Chronic disabling postpartum headache after unintentional dural puncture during epidural anaesthesia: a prospective cohort study. Br J Anaesth 2021;Clinical Investigation/Articles in Press.

5. Attanasio L, Kozhimannil KB, Jou J, et al. Women's Experiences with Neuraxial Labor Analgesia in the Listening to Mothers II Survey: A Content Analysis of Open-Ended Responses. Anesth Analg 2015;121(4):974-80.

6. Bannister-Tyrrell M, Ford JB, Morris JM, et al. Epidural analgesia in labour and risk of caesarean delivery. Paediatr Perinat Epidemiol 2014;28(5):400-11.

7. Bannister-Tyrrell M, Miladinovic B, Roberts CL, et al. Adjustment for compliance behavior in trials of epidural analgesia in labor using instrumental variable meta-analysis. J Clin Epidemiol 2015;68(5):525-33.

8. Behrens O, Goeschen K, Luck HJ, et al. Effects of lumbar epidural analgesia on prostaglandin F2 alpha release and oxytocin secretion during labor. Prostaglandins 1993;45(3):285-96.

9. Beilin Y, Bodian CA, Weiser J, et al. Effect of labor epidural analgesia with and without fentanyl on infant breast-feeding: a prospective, randomized, double-blind study. Anesthesiology 2005;103(6):1211-7.

10. Beilin Y, Friedman F, Jr., Andres LA, et al. The effect of the obstetrician group and epidural analgesia on the risk for cesarean delivery in nulliparous women. Acta Anaesthesiol Scand 2000;44(8):959-64.

11. Benaron DA. Subgaleal hematoma causing hypovolemic shock during delivery after failed vacuum extraction: a case report. J Perinatol 1993;13(3):228-31.

12. Bernitz S, Oian P, Rolland R, et al. Oxytocin and dystocia as risk factors for adverse birth outcomes: a cohort of low-risk nulliparous women. Midwifery 2014;30(3):364-70.

13. Blanks AM, Shmygol A, Thornton S. Regulation of oxytocin receptors and oxytocin receptor signaling. Semin Reprod Med 2007;25(1):52-9.

14. Block J. Pushed: The Painful Truth About Childbirth and Modern Maternity Care. Cambridge, MA: Da Capo Press; 2007.

15. Here's what it costs to actually become a mother. Money, May 6, 2016. (Accessed Apr 21, 2021, at https://money.com/childbirth-cost-insurance-mother/.)

16. Brimdyr K, Cadwell K, Widstrom AM, et al. The association between common labor drugs and suckling when skin-to-skin during the first hour after birth. Birth 2015;42(4):319-28.

17. Brimdyr K, Cadwell K, Widstrom AM, et al. The effect of labor medications on normal newborn behavior in the first hour after birth: A prospective cohort study. Early Hum Dev 2019;132:30-6.

18. Buckley SJ. Hormonal physiology of childbearing: Evidence and implications for women, babies, and maternity care. Washington, D.C.; 2015.

19. Chantry CJ, Nommsen-Rivers LA, Peerson JM, et al. Excess Weight Loss in First-Born Breastfed Newborns Relates to Maternal Intrapartum Fluid Balance. Pediatrics 2011;127(1):171-9.

20. Cheng YW, Shaffer BL, Caughey AB. Associated factors and outcomes of persistent occiput posterior position: A retrospective cohort study from 1976 to 2001. J Matern Fetal Neonatal Med 2006;19(9):563-8.

21. Chua K, Fendrick AM, Conti RM, et al. Prevalence and magnitude of potential surprise bills for childbirth. JAMA Health Forum 2021;2(7):e211460.

22. Declercq E, Sakala C, Corry MP, et al. Listening to Mothers II: Report of the Second National U.S. Survey of Women's Childbearing Experiences. New York: Childbirth Connection; 2006.

23. Dozier AM, Howard CR, Brownell EA, et al. Labor epidural anesthesia, obstetric factors and breastfeeding cessation. Matern Child Health J 2013;17(4):689-98.

24. Eriksen LM, Nohr EA, Kjaergaard H. Mode of delivery after epidural analgesia in a cohort of low-risk nulliparas. Birth 2011;38(4):317-26.

25. Fernando R, Bonello E, Gill P, et al. Neonatal welfare and placental transfer of fentanyl and bupivacaine during ambulatory combined spinal epidural analgesia for labour. Anaesthesia 1997;52(6):517-24.

26. Fitzpatrick M, McQuillan K, O'Herlihy C. Influence of persistent occiput posterior position on delivery outcome. Obstet Gynecol 2001;98(6):1027-31.

27. French CA, Cong X, Chung KS. Labor Epidural Analgesia and Breast-feeding: A Systematic Review. J Hum Lact 2016;32(3):507-20.

28. Gizzo S, Di Gangi S, Noventa M, et al. Women's choice of positions during labour: return to the past or a modern way to give birth? A cohort study in Italy. Biomed Res Int 2014:638093.

29. Green JM. Expectations and experiences of pain in labor: findings from a large prospective study. Birth 1993;20(2):65-72.

30. Guillemette J, Fraser WD. Differences between obstetricians in caesarean section rates and the management of labour. Br J Obstet Gynaecol 1992;99(2):105-8.

31. Henderson JJ, Dickinson JE, Evans SF, et al. Impact of intrapartum epidural analgesia on breast-feeding duration. Aust N Z J Obstet Gynaecol 2003;43(5):372-7.

32. Hoefnagel A, Yu A, Kaminski A. Anesthetic Complications in Pregnancy. Crit Care Clin 2016;32(1):1-28.

33. Jansen S, Lopriore E, Naaktgeboren C, et al. Epidural-Related Fever and Maternal and Neonatal Morbidity: A Systematic Review and Meta-Analysis. Neonatology 2020;117(3):259-70.

34. Janssen PA, Klein MC, Soolsma JH. Differences in institutional cesarean delivery rates—the role of pain management. J Fam Pract 2001;50(3):217-23.

35. Jonas K, Johansson LM, Nissen E, et al. Effects of intrapartum oxytocin administration and epidural analgesia on the concentration of plasma oxytocin and prolactin, in response to suckling during the second day postpartum. Breastfeed Med 2009;4(2):71-82.

36. Jordan S, Emery S, Bradshaw C, et al. The impact of intrapartum analgesia on infant feeding. BJOG 2005;112(7):927-34.

37. Klein MC, Grzybowski S, Harris S, et al. Epidural analgesia use as a marker for physician approach to birth: implications for maternal and newborn outcomes. Birth 2001;28(4):243-8.

38. Klomp T, van Poppel M, Jones L, et al. Inhaled analgesia for pain management in labour. Cochrane Database Syst Rev 2012;9:CD009351.

39. Lawrence A, Lewis L, Hofmeyr GJ, et al. Maternal positions and mobility during first stage labour. Cochrane Database Syst Rev 2013;10:CD003934.

40. Lieberman E, Davidson K, Lee-Parritz A, et al. Changes in fetal position during labor and their association with epidural analgesia. Obstet Gynecol 2005;105(5 Pt 1):974-82.

41. Lieberman E, O'Donoghue C. Unintended effects of epidural analgesia during labor: a systematic review. Am J Obstet Gynecol 2002;186(5 Suppl Nature):S31-68.

42. Likis FE, Andrews JC, Collins MR, et al. Nitrous oxide for the management of labor pain: a systematic review. Anesth Analg 2014;118(1):153-67.

43. Lind JN, Perrine CG, Li R. Relationship between use of labor pain medications and delayed onset of lactation. J Hum Lact 2014;30(2):167-73.

44. Loftus JR, Hill H, Cohen SE. Placental transfer and neonatal effects of epidural sufentanil and fentanyl administered with bupivacaine during labor. Anesthesiology 1995;83(2):300-8.

45. Mackenzie M. Should you get a C-section? Redbook 2016 Oct 21, 2016.

46. Magann EF, Evans S, Hutchinson M, et al. Postpartum hemorrhage after vaginal birth: an analysis of risk factors. South Med J 2005;98(4):419-22.

47. Mardirosoff C, Dumont L, Boulvain M, et al. Fetal bradycardia due to intrathecal opioids for labour analgesia: a systematic review. BJOG 2002;109(3):274-81.

48. Martens PJ, Romphf L. Factors associated with newborn in-hospital weight loss: comparisons by feeding method, demographics, and birthing procedures. J Hum Lact 2007;23(3):233-41, quiz 42-5.

49. Morton S, Kua J, Mullington CJ. Epidural analgesia, intrapartum hyperthermia, and neonatal brain injury: a systematic review and meta-analysis. Br J Anaesth 2021;126(2):500-15.

50. Nguyen US, Rothman KJ, Demissie S, et al. Epidural analgesia and risks of cesarean and operative vaginal deliveries in nulliparous and multiparous women. Matern Child Health J 2010;14(5):705-12.

51. Niraj G, Mushambi M, Gauthama P, et al. Persistent headache and low back pain after accidental dural puncture in the obstetric population: a prospective, observational, multicentre cohort study. Anaesthesia 2021;76(8):1068-76.

52. Paech MJ, Godkin R, Webster S. Complications of obstetric epidural analgesia and anaesthesia: a prospective analysis of 10,995 cases. Int J Obstet Anesth 1998;7(1):5-11.

53. Ponkey SE, Cohen AP, Heffner LJ, et al. Persistent fetal occiput posterior position: obstetric outcomes. Obstet Gynecol 2003;101(5 Pt 1):915-20.

54. Public Health Agency of Canada. What Mothers Say: The Canadian Maternity Experiences Survey. Ottawa; 2009.

55. Rahm VA, Hallgren A, Hogberg H, et al. Plasma oxytocin levels in women during labor with or without epidural analgesia: a prospective study. Acta Obstet Gynecol Scand 2002;81(11):1033-9.

56. Ranganathan P, Golfeiz C, Phelps AL, et al. Chronic headache and backache are long-term sequelae of unintentional dural puncture in the obstetric population. J Clin Anesth 2015;27(3):201-6.

57. Ravelli ACJ, Eskes M, de Groot CJM, et al. Intrapartum epidural analgesia and low Apgar score among singleton infants born at term: A propensity score matched study. Acta Obstet Gynecol Scand 2020;99(9):1155-62.

58. Reynolds F, Laishley R, Morgan B, et al. Effect of time and adrenaline on the feto-maternal distribution of bupivacaine. Br J Anaesth 1989;62(5):509-14.

59. Why is oxytocin known as the "love hormone"? And 11 other FAQs. Healthline, Aug 30, 2018. (Accessed Apr 21, 2021, at https://www.healthline.com/health/love-hormone.)

60. Scott DB, Tunstall ME. Serious complications associated with epidural/spinal blockade in obstetrics: a two-year prospective study. Int J Obstet Anesth 1995;4(3):133-9.

61. Segal S, Blatman R, Doble M, et al. The influence of the obstetrician in the relationship between epidural analgesia and cesarean section for dystocia. Anesthesiology 1999;91(1):90-6.

62. Shmueli A, Salman L, Orbach-Zinger S, et al. The impact of epidural analgesia on the duration of the second stage of labor. Birth 2018;45(4):377-84.

63. Simkin P. Moving beyond the debate: a holistic approach to understanding and treating effects of neuraxial analgesia. Birth 2012;39(4):327-32.

64. Sizer AR, Nirmal DM. Occipitoposterior position: associated factors and obstetric outcome in nulliparas. Obstet Gynecol 2000;96(5 Pt 1):749-52.

65. Smith LA, Burns E, Cuthbert A. Parenteral opioids for maternal pain management in labour. Cochrane Database Syst Rev 2018;6:CD007396.

66. Thomson G, Feeley C, Moran VH, et al. Women's experiences of pharmacological and non-pharmacological pain relief methods for labour and childbirth: a qualitative systematic review. Reprod Health 2019;16(1):71.

67. Tingaker BK, Irestedt L. Changes in uterine innervation in pregnancy and during labour. Curr Opin Anaesthesiol 2010;23(3):300-3.

68. Torvaldsen S, Roberts CL, Simpson JM, et al. Intrapartum epidural analgesia and breastfeeding: a prospective cohort study. Int Breastfeed J 2006;1:24.

69. Villarosa L. Making an appointment with the stork. New York Times Jun 23, 2002.

70. Wang F, Shen X, Guo X, et al. Epidural analgesia in the latent phase of labor and the risk of cesarean delivery: a five-year randomized controlled trial. Anesthesiology 2009;111(4):871-80.

71. Webb CA, Weyker PD, Zhang L, et al. Unintentional dural puncture with a Tuohy needle increases risk of chronic headache. Anesth Analg 2012;115(1):124-32.

72. The high U.S. c-section rate could endanger lives. 2016. (Accessed Jan 13, 2016, at http://thefederalist.com/2016/01/13/the-high-u-s-c-section-rate-could-endanger-lives/.)

73. Breastfeeding and antibiotics: What you need to know. Healthline Parenthood, June 17, 2020. (Accessed Apr 4, 2021, at https://www.healthline.com/health/breastfeeding/breastfeeding-and-antibiotics.)

CHAPTER 3: COMBINED SPINAL-EPIDURALS

1. Albright GA, Forster RM. The safety and efficacy of combined spinal and epidural analgesia/anesthesia (6,002 blocks) in a community hospital. Reg Anesth Pain Med 1999;24(2):117-25.

2. COMET Study Group. Effect of low-dose mobile versus traditional epidural techniques on mode of delivery: a randomised controlled trial. Lancet 2001;358(9275):19-23.

3. Friedlander JD, Fox HE, Cain CF, et al. Fetal bradycardia and uterine hyperactivity following subarachnoid administration of fentanyl during labor. Reg Anesth 1997;22(4):378-81.

4. Gambling DR, Sharma SK, Ramin SM, et al. A randomized study of combined spinal-epidural analgesia versus intravenous meperidine during labor: impact on cesarean delivery rate. Anesthesiology 1998;89(6):1336-44.

5. Grangier L, Martinez de Tejada B, Savoldelli GL, et al. Adverse side effects and route of administration of opioids in combined spinal-epidural analgesia for labour: a meta-analysis of randomised trials. Int J Obstet Anesth 2020;41:83-103.

6. Hattler J, Klimek M, Rossaint R, et al. The Effect of Combined Spinal-Epidural Versus Epidural Analgesia in Laboring Women on Nonreassuring Fetal Heart Rate Tracings: Systematic Review and Meta-analysis. Anesth Analg 2016;123(4):955-64.

7. Katsiris S, Williams S, Leighton BL, et al. Respiratory arrest following intrathecal injection of sufentanil and bupivacaine in a parturient. Can J Anaesth 1998;45(9):880-3.

8. Kehl F, Erfkamp S, Roewer N. Respiratory arrest during caesarean section after intrathecal administration of sufentanil in combination with 0.1% bupivacaine 10 ml. Anaesth Intensive Care 2002;30(5):698-9.

9. Klein M. Personal Communication re Administration of a combined spinal-epidural. In: Goer H, ed.; 2021.

10. Kuczkowski KM. Respiratory arrest in a parturient following intrathecal administration of fentanyl and bupivacaine as part of a combined spinal-epidural analgesia for labour. Anaesthesia 2002;57(9):939-40.

11. Kuczkowski KM. Severe persistent fetal bradycardia following subarachnoid administration of fentanyl and bupivacaine for induction of a combined spinal-epidural analgesia for labor pain. J Clin Anesth 2004;16(1):78-9.

12. Nielsen PE, Erickson JR, Abouleish EI, et al. Fetal heart rate changes after intrathecal sufentanil or epidural bupivacaine for labor analgesia: incidence and clinical significance. Anesth Analg 1996;83(4):742-6.

13. Sachs A, Smiley R. Post-dural puncture headache: the worst common complication in obstetric anesthesia. Semin Perinatol 2014;38(6):386-94.

14. Simmons SW, Taghizadeh N, Dennis AT, et al. Combined spinal-epidural versus epidural analgesia in labour. Cochrane Database Syst Rev 2012;10:CD003401.

CHAPTER 4: OPIOIDS

1. Anim-Somuah M, Smyth RM, Cyna AM, et al. Epidural versus non-epidural or no analgesia for pain management in labour. Cochrane Database Syst Rev 2018;5:CD000331.

2. Bai DL, Wu KM, Tarrant M. Association between intrapartum interventions and breastfeeding duration. J Midwifery Womens Health 2013;58(1):25-32.

3. Here's what it costs to actually become a mother. Money, May 6, 2016. (Accessed Apr 21, 2021, at https://money.com/childbirth-cost-insurance-mother/.)

4. Buckley SJ. Hormonal physiology of childbearing: Evidence and implications for women, babies, and maternity care. Washington, D.C.; 2015.

5. Chua K, Fendrick AM, Conti RM, et al. Prevalence and magnitude of potential surprise bills for childbirth. JAMA Health Forum 2021;2(7):e211460.

6. Declercq E, Sakala C, Corry MP, et al. Listening to Mothers II: Report of the Second National U.S. Survey of Women's Childbearing Experiences. New York: Childbirth Connection; 2006.

7. Henderson JJ, Dickinson JE, Evans SF, et al. Impact of intrapartum epidural analgesia on breast-feeding duration. Aust N Z J Obstet Gynaecol 2003;43(5):372-7.

8. Klomp T, van Poppel M, Jones L, et al. Inhaled analgesia for pain management in labour. Cochrane Database Syst Rev 2012;9:CD009351.

9. Likis FE, Andrews JC, Collins MR, et al. Nitrous oxide for the management of labor pain: a systematic review. Anesth Analg 2014;118(1):153-67.

10. Lind JN, Perrine CG, Li R. Relationship between use of labor pain medications and delayed onset of lactation. J Hum Lact 2014;30(2):167-73.

11. Mardirosoff C, Dumont L, Boulvain M, et al. Fetal bradycardia due to intrathecal opioids for labour analgesia: a systematic review. BJOG 2002;109(3):274-81.

12. Nethery E, Schummers L, Levine A, et al. Birth Outcomes for Planned Home and Licensed Freestanding Birth Center Births in Washington State. Obstet Gynecol 2021;138(5):693-702.

13. Public Health Agency of Canada. What Mothers Say: The Canadian Maternity Experiences Survey. Ottawa; 2009.

14. Why is oxytocin known as the "love hormone"? And 11 other FAQs. Healthline, Aug 30, 2018. (Accessed Apr 21, 2021, at https://www.healthline.com/health/love-hormone.)

15. Smith LA, Burns E, Cuthbert A. Parenteral opioids for maternal pain management in labour. Cochrane Database Syst Rev 2018;6:CD007396.

16. Thomson G, Feeley C, Moran VH, et al. Women's experiences of pharmacological and non-pharmacological pain relief methods for labour and childbirth: a qualitative systematic review. Reprod Health 2019;16(1):71.

17. Torvaldsen S, Roberts CL, Simpson JM, et al. Intrapartum epidural analgesia and breastfeeding: a prospective cohort study. Int Breastfeed J 2006;1:24.

18. Wee MY, Tuckey JP, Thomas PW, et al. A comparison of intramuscular diamorphine and intramuscular pethidine for labour analgesia: a two-centre randomised blinded controlled trial. BJOG 2014;121(4):447-56.

19. Weibel S, Jelting Y, Afshari A, et al. Patient-controlled analgesia with remifentanil versus alternative parenteral methods for pain management in labour. Cochrane Database Syst Rev 2017;4:CD011989.

20. Wilson MJ, MacArthur C, Cooper GM, et al. Epidural analgesia and breastfeeding: a randomised controlled trial of epidural techniques with and without fentanyl and a non-epidural comparison group. Anaesthesia 2010;65(2):145-53.

CHAPTER 5: NITROUS OXIDE

1. Here's what it costs to actually become a mother. Money, May 6, 2016. (Accessed Apr 21, 2021, at https://money.com/childbirth-cost-insurance-mother/.)

2. Laughing gas is now an option for women in labor. People.com, Jan 23, 2015. (Accessed Dec 14, 2015, at https://people.com/celebrity/laughing-gas-for-women-in-labor/.)

3. Chua K, Fendrick AM, Conti RM, et al. Prevalence and magnitude of potential surprise bills for childbirth. JAMA Health Forum 2021;2(7):e211460.

4. Dammer U, Weiss C, Raabe E, et al. Introduction of Inhaled Nitrous Oxide and Oxygen for Pain Management during Labour - Evaluation of Patients' and Midwives' Satisfaction. Geburtshilfe Frauenheilkd 2014;74(7):656-60.

5. Gizzo S, Di Gangi S, Noventa M, et al. Women's choice of positions during labour: return to the past or a modern way to give birth? A cohort study in Italy. Biomed Res Int 2014;2014:638093.

6. Klomp T, van Poppel M, Jones L, et al. Inhaled analgesia for pain management in labour. Cochrane Database Syst Rev 2012;9:CD009351.

7. Lawrence A, Lewis L, Hofmeyr GJ, et al. Maternal positions and mobility during first stage labour. Cochrane Database Syst Rev 2013;10:CD003934.

8. Likis FE, Andrews JC, Collins MR, et al. Nitrous oxide for the management of labor pain: a systematic review. Anesth Analg 2014;118(1):153-67.

9. The Birthplace offers nitrous oxide for pain relief in labor. The Recorder, Mar 5, 2015. (Accessed Mar 6, 2015, at [article archived behind a paywall].)

10. Nodine PM, Collins MR, Wood CL, et al. Nitrous Oxide Use During Labor: Satisfaction, Adverse Effects, and Predictors of Conversion to Neuraxial Analgesia. J Midwifery Womens Health 2020;65(3):335-41.

11. Richardson MG, Raymond BL, Baysinger CL, et al. A qualitative analysis of parturients' experiences using nitrous oxide for labor analgesia: It is not just about pain relief. Birth 2019;46(1):97-104.

12. Smith LA, Burns E, Cuthbert A. Parenteral opioids for mater-
    nal pain management in labour. Cochrane Database Syst Rev
    2018;6:CD007396.

13. Weibel S, Jelting Y, Afshari A, et al. Patient-controlled analgesia with
    remifentanil versus alternative parenteral methods for pain management
    in labour. Cochrane Database Syst Rev 2017;4:CD011989.

CHAPTER 6: DIY STRATEGIES

1. Bayes S, Fenwick J, Hauck Y. A qualitative analysis of women's short
   accounts of labour and birth in a Western Australian public tertiary
   hospital. J Midwifery Womens Health 2008;53(1):53-61.

2. Bohren MA, Hofmeyr GJ, Sakala C, et al. Continuous support for women during childbirth. Cochrane Database Syst Rev
   2017;7:CD003766.

3. Bovbjerg ML, Cheyney M, Everson C. Maternal and Newborn Outcomes Following Waterbirth: The Midwives Alliance of North America
   Statistics Project, 2004 to 2009 Cohort. J Midwifery Womens Health
   2016;61(1):11-20.

4. Bowers BB. Mothers' experiences of labor support: exploration of qualitative research. J Obstet Gynecol Neonatal Nurs 2002;31(6):742-52.

5. Chaillet N, Belaid L, Crochetiere C, et al. Nonpharmacologic ap-
   proaches for pain management during labor compared with usual care:
   a meta-analysis. Birth 2014;41(2):122-37.

6. Christiaens W, Bracke P. Assessment of social psychological determi-
   nants of satisfaction with childbirth in a cross-national perspective.
   BMC Pregnancy Childbirth 2007;7:26.

7. Cluett ER, Burns E, Cuthbert A. Immersion in water during labour and
   birth. Cochrane Database Syst Rev 2018;5:CD000111.

8. Cooper M, Warland J. What are the benefits? Are they concerned?
   Women's experiences of water immersion for labor and birth. Midwifery
   2019;79:102541.

9. Davis E, Pascali-Bonaro D. Orgasmic Birth: Your Guide to a Safe,
   Satisfying, and Pleasureable Birth Experience: Rodale Press; 2010.

10. Declercq E, Sakala C, Corry MP, et al. Listening to Mothers II: Report of the Second National U.S. Survey of Women's Childbearing Experiences. New York: Childbirth Connection; 2006.

11. Feeley C, Cooper M, Burns E. A systematic meta-thematic synthesis to examine the views and experiences of women following water immersion during labour and waterbirth. J Adv Nurs 2021;77(7):2942-56.

12. Goodman P, Mackey MC, Tavakoli AS. Factors related to childbirth satisfaction. J Adv Nurs 2004;46(2):212-9.

13. Green JM. Expectations and experiences of pain in labor: findings from a large prospective study. Birth 1993;20(2):65-72.

14. Hardin AM, Buckner EB. Characteristics of a positive experience for women who have unmedicated childbirth. J Perinat Educ 2004;13(4):10-6.

15. Jones L, Othman M, Dowswell T, et al. Pain management for women in labour: an overview of systematic reviews. Cochrane Database Syst Rev 2012;3:CD009234.

16. Lee SL, Liu CY, Lu YY, et al. Efficacy of warm showers on labor pain and birth experiences during the first labor stage. J Obstet Gynecol Neonatal Nurs 2013;42(1):19-28.

17. Levett KM, Smith CA, Bensoussan A, et al. Complementary therapies for labour and birth study: a randomised controlled trial of antenatal integrative medicine for pain management in labour. BMJ Open 2016;6(7):e010691.

18. Lukasse M, Rowe R, Townend J, et al. Immersion in water for pain relief and the risk of intrapartum transfer among low risk nulliparous women: secondary analysis of the Birthplace national prospective cohort study. BMC Pregnancy Childbirth 2014;14:60.

19. Melender HL. What constitutes a good childbirth? A qualitative study of pregnant Finnish women. J Midwifery Womens Health 2006;51(5):331-9.

20. Mozingo JN, Davis MW, Thomas SP, et al. "I felt violated": women's experience of childbirth-associated anger. MCN Am J Matern Child Nurs 2002;27(6):342-8.

21. Public Health Agency of Canada. What Mothers Say: The Canadian Maternity Experiences Survey. Ottawa; 2009.

22. Rijnders M, Baston H, Schonbeck Y, et al. Perinatal factors related to negative or positive recall of birth experience in women 3 years postpartum in the Netherlands. Birth 2008;35(2):107-16.

23. Siegel P. Does bath water enter the vagina? Obstet Gynecol 1960;15:660-1.

24. Simkin P. Just another day in a woman's life? Women's long-term perceptions of their first birth experience. Part I. Birth 1991;18(4):203-10.

25. Snapp C, Stapleton SR, Wright J, et al. The Experience of Land and Water Birth Within the American Association of Birth Centers Perinatal Data Registry, 2012-2017. J Perinat Neonatal Nurs 2020;34(1):16-26.

26. Thomson G, Feeley C, Moran VH, et al. Women's experiences of pharmacological and non-pharmacological pain relief methods for labour and childbirth: a qualitative systematic review. Reprod Health 2019;16(1):71.

27. Veringa-Skiba IK, de Bruin EI, van Steensel FJA, et al. Fear of childbirth, nonurgent obstetric interventions, and newborn outcomes: A randomized controlled trial comparing mindfulness-based childbirth and parenting with enhanced care as usual. Birth 2021.

28. Waldenstrom U, Hildingsson I, Rubertsson C, et al. A negative birth experience: prevalence and risk factors in a national sample. Birth 2004;31(1):17-27.

29. Whitburn LY, Jones LE, Davey MA, et al. The meaning of labour pain: how the social environment and other contextual factors shape women's experiences. BMC Pregnancy Childbirth 2017;17(1):157.

CHAPTER 7: YOUR TAKE-AWAY

1. Albright GA, Forster RM. The safety and efficacy of combined spinal and epidural analgesia/anesthesia (6,002 blocks) in a community hospital. Reg Anesth Pain Med 1999;24(2):117-25.

2. Bernitz S, Oian P, Rolland R, et al. Oxytocin and dystocia as risk factors for adverse birth outcomes: a cohort of low-risk nulliparous women. Midwifery 2014;30(3):364-70.

3. Block J. Pushed: The Painful Truth About Childbirth and Modern Maternity Care. Cambridge, MA: Da Capo Press; 2007.

4. Here's what it costs to actually become a mother. Money, May 6, 2016. (Accessed Apr 21, 2021, at https://money.com/childbirth-cost-insurance-mother/.)

5. Brimdyr K, Cadwell K, Widstrom AM, et al. The association between common labor drugs and suckling when skin-to-skin during the first hour after birth. Birth 2015;42(4):319-28.

6. Carlton T, Callister LC, Christiaens G, et al. Labor and delivery nurses' perceptions of caring for childbearing women in nurse-managed birthing units. MCN Am J Matern Child Nurs 2009;34(1):50-6.

7. Carlton T, Callister LC, Stoneman E. Decision making in laboring women: ethical issues for perinatal nurses. J Perinat Neonatal Nurs 2005;19(2):145-54.

8. Cheng YW, Shaffer BL, Nicholson JM, et al. Second stage of labor and epidural use: a larger effect than previously suggested. Obstet Gynecol 2014;123(3):527-35.

9. Chua K, Fendrick AM, Conti RM, et al. Prevalence and magnitude of potential surprise bills for childbirth. JAMA Health Forum 2021;2(7):e211460.

10. Davies BL, Hodnett E. Labor support: nurses' self-efficacy and views about factors influencing implementation. J Obstet Gynecol Neonatal Nurs 2002;31(1):48-56.

11. Declercq E, Sakala C, Corry MP, et al. Listening to Mothers II: Report of the Second National U.S. Survey of Women's Childbearing Experiences. New York: Childbirth Connection; 2006.

12. Declercq E, Sakala C, Corry MP, et al. Listening to Mothers III: New Mothers Speak Out. New York: Childbirth Connection; 2013.

13. Dozier AM, Howard CR, Brownell EA, et al. Labor epidural anesthesia, obstetric factors and breastfeeding cessation. Matern Child Health J 2013;17(4):689-98.

14. Gagnon AJ, Waghorn K. Supportive care by maternity nurses: a work sampling study in an intrapartum unit. Birth 1996;23(1):1-6.

15. Gale J, Fothergill-Bourbonnais F, Chamberlain M. Measuring nursing support during childbirth. MCN Am J Matern Child Nurs 2001;26(5):264-71.

16. Goer H. Dueling cesarean statistics: What should the cesarean rate be? — Henci Goer compares recent studies. In: Muza S, ed. Science and Sensibility: Lamaze International; 2015.

17. Goer H. Epidural analgesia: To delay or not to delay, that is the question. In: Muza S, ed. Science and Sensibility: Lamaze Inernational; Oct 23, 2014.

18. Goldberg HB, Shorten A. Patient and provider perceptions of decision making about use of epidural analgesia during childbirth: a thematic analysis. J Perinat Educ 2014;23(3):142-50.

19. Green JM. Expectations and experiences of pain in labor: findings from a large prospective study. Birth 1993;20(2):65-72.

20. Halpern SH, Levine T, Wilson DB, et al. Effect of labor analgesia on breastfeeding success. Birth 1999;26(2):83-8.

21. Hoefnagel A, Yu A, Kaminski A. Anesthetic Complications in Pregnancy. Crit Care Clin 2016;32(1):1-28.

22. Klein MC. Does epidural analgesia increase rate of cesarean section? Can Fam Physician 2006;52:419-21, 26-8.

23. Knox A, Rouleau G, Semenic S, et al. Barriers and facilitators to birth without epidural in a tertiary obstetric referral center: Perspectives of health care professionals and patients. Birth 2018;45(3):295-302.

24. Leeman L, Fontaine P, King V, et al. Management of labor pain: promoting patient choice. Am Fam Physician 2003;68(6):1023, 6, 33 passim.

25. Lieberman E, Lang JM, Cohen A, et al. Association of epidural analgesia with cesarean delivery in nulliparas. Obstet Gynecol 1996;88(6):993-1000.

26. Lieberman E, O'Donoghue C. Unintended effects of epidural analgesia during labor: a systematic review. Am J Obstet Gynecol 2002;186(5 Suppl Nature):S31-68.

27. McNiven P, Hodnett E, O'Brien-Pallas LL. Supporting women in labor: a work sampling study of the activities of labor and delivery nurses. Birth 1992;19(1):3-8; discussion 8-9.

28. Miltner RS. More than support: nursing interventions provided to women in labor. J Obstet Gynecol Neonatal Nurs 2002;31(6):753-61.

29. Morell E, Peralta FM, Higgins N, et al. Effect of companion presence on maternal satisfaction during neuraxial catheter placement for labor analgesia: a randomized clinical trial. Int J Obstet Anesth 2019;38:66-74.

30. Niraj G, Mushambi M, Gauthama P, et al. Persistent headache and low back pain after accidental dural puncture in the obstetric population: a prospective, observational, multicentre cohort study. Anaesthesia 2021;76(8):1068-76.

31. Nodine PM, Collins MR, Wood CL, et al. Nitrous Oxide Use During Labor: Satisfaction, Adverse Effects, and Predictors of Conversion to Neuraxial Analgesia. J Midwifery Womens Health 2020;65(3):335-41.

32. Papagni K, Buckner E. Doula Support and Attitudes of Intrapartum Nurses: A Qualitative Study from the Patient's Perspective. J Perinat Educ 2006;15(1):11-8.

33. Payant L, Davies B, Graham ID, et al. Nurses' intentions to provide continuous labor support to women. J Obstet Gynecol Neonatal Nurs 2008;37(4):405-14.

34. Public Health Agency of Canada. What Mothers Say: The Canadian Maternity Experiences Survey. Ottawa; 2009.

35. Radzyminski S. The effect of ultra low dose epidural analgesia on newborn breastfeeding behaviors. J Obstet Gynecol Neonatal Nurs 2003;32(3):322-31.

36. Richardson MG, Raymond BL, Baysinger CL, et al. A qualitative analysis of parturients' experiences using nitrous oxide for labor analgesia: It is not just about pain relief. Birth 2019;46(1):97-104.

37. Sakala C, Declercq E, Turon JM, et al. Listening to Mothers in California. Washington, D.C.: National Partnership for Women & Families; 2018.

38. Simkin P. Moving beyond the debate: a holistic approach to understanding and treating effects of neuraxial analgesia. Birth 2012;39(4):327-32.

39. Simkin P, Hanson L, Ancheta R. The Labor Progress Handbook. Hoboken, NJ: Wiley-Blackwell; 2017.

40. Simmonds AH, Peter E, Hodnett ED, et al. Understanding the moral nature of intrapartum nursing. J Obstet Gynecol Neonatal Nurs 2013;42(2):148-56.

41. Sleutel M, Schultz S, Wyble K. Nurses' views of factors that help and hinder their intrapartum care. J Obstet Gynecol Neonatal Nurs 2007;36(3):203-11.

42. Sng BL, Leong WL, Zeng Y, et al. Early versus late initiation of epidural analgesia for labour. Cochrane Database Syst Rev 2014;10:CD007238.

43. Thomson G, Feeley C, Moran VH, et al. Women's experiences of pharmacological and non-pharmacological pain relief methods for labour and childbirth: a qualitative systematic review. Reprod Health 2019;16(1):71.

44. Thorp JA, Hu DH, Albin RM, et al. The effect of intrapartum epidural analgesia on nulliparous labor: a randomized, controlled, prospective trial. Am J Obstet Gynecol 1993;169(4):851-8.

45. Webb CA, Weyker PD, Zhang L, et al. Unintentional dural puncture with a Tuohy needle increases risk of chronic headache. Anesth Analg 2012;115(1):124-32.

46. Weibel S, Jelting Y, Afshari A, et al. Patient-controlled analgesia with remifentanil versus alternative parenteral methods for pain management in labour. Cochrane Database Syst Rev 2017;4:CD011989.

47. Whitburn LY, Jones LE, Davey MA, et al. The meaning of labour pain: how the social environment and other contextual factors shape women's experiences. BMC Pregnancy Childbirth 2017;17(1):157.

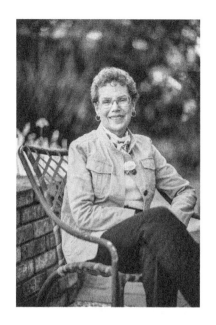

S tarting out as a Lamaze teacher and doula, Henci Goer's life's work soon became analyzing and synthesizing the obstetric research in order to give pregnant women and birth professionals access to what constitutes optimal care in childbirth.

She is the author of three books: *Optimal Care in Childbirth: The Case for a Physiologic Approach* (co-author Amy Romano MSN, CNM), *The Thinking Woman's Guide to a Better Birth*, and *Obstetric Myths Versus Research Realities*. In addition, she has written numerous blog posts and articles and given lectures around the world.

In recognition of her work, she has received, among others, the American College of Nurse-Midwives Best Book of the Year Award, Lamaze International's President's Award, DONA International's Klaus & Kennell Research Award, a Lifetime Achievement Award from BOLD Atlanta, and the Media Award from the American Association of Birth Centers.

The "Take Charge of Your Birth" series—short books on single topics to help women make informed choices and obtain optimal care for themselves and their babies—is a continuation of her work.

For more about Henci's work, visit www.HenciGoer.com.

For more childbirth research and the latest news, sign up at

www.hencigoer.com/newsletter

Made in the USA
Monee, IL
17 August 2023

41114979R00089